D0322975

Premature Infants and Their Families
Developmental Interventions

25K.
WYL.

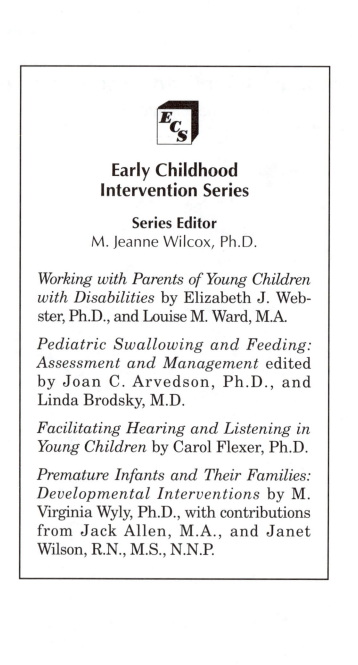

**Early Childhood
Intervention Series**

Series Editor
M. Jeanne Wilcox, Ph.D.

*Working with Parents of Young Children
with Disabilities* by Elizabeth J. Web-
ster, Ph.D., and Louise M. Ward, M.A.

*Pediatric Swallowing and Feeding:
Assessment and Management* edited
by Joan C. Arvedson, Ph.D., and
Linda Brodsky, M.D.

*Facilitating Hearing and Listening in
Young Children* by Carol Flexer, Ph.D.

*Premature Infants and Their Families:
Developmental Interventions* by M.
Virginia Wyly, Ph.D., with contributions
from Jack Allen, M.A., and Janet
Wilson, R.N., M.S., N.N.P.

Premature Infants and Their Families
Developmental Interventions

By

M. Virginia Wyly, Ph.D.
Buffalo State College
State University of New York
with contributions from
Jack Allen, M.A.
and
Janet Wilson, R.N., M.S., N.N.P.

WITHDRAWN

Singular Publishing Group, Inc.
San Diego · London

618. 92011 WYL

Singular Publishing Group, Inc.
4284 41st Street
San Diego, California 92105-1197

19 Compton Terrace
London, N1 2UN, UK

© **1995 by Singular Publishing Group, Inc.**

Typeset in 10/12 New Century Schoolbook by So Cal Graphics

Printed in the United States of America by McNaughton & Gunn

All rights, including that of translation reserved. No part of this publication may be reproduced, stored in a retrieval system, or transmitted in any form or by any means, electronic, mechanical, recording, or otherwise, without the prior written permission of the publisher.

Library of Congress Cataloging-in-Publication Data

Wyly, M. Virginia (Mary Virginia)
   Premature infants and their families : developmental interventions /
   by M. Virginia Wyly, with contributions from Jack Allen ... [et al.].
     p. cm.—(Early childhood intervention series)
   Includes bibliographical references and index.
   ISBN 1-879105-87-X
   1. Infants (Premature) 2. Neonatal intensive care. 3. Infants
(Premature)—Family relationships. I. Title. II. Series.
   [DNLM: 1. Infant, Premature. 2. Neonatal Nursing—methods.
   3. Intensive Care Units, Neonatal. 4. Family—psychology.
   5. Caregivers. WS 410 W983p   1995]
RJ250.W95 1995
618.92'011—dc20
DNLM/DLC
for Library of Congress
                                                  95–271
                                                     CIP

Contents

■

Foreword

When current social policy regarding at-risk infants and young children is considered in conjunction with advances in theoretical conceptualizations and associated research it is clear that early childhood intervention is emerging as a unique and dynamic area of scientific inquiry across multiple disciplines. The purpose of the *Early Childhood Intervention Series* is to provide state-of-the-art information with respect to interventions focusing on families and their infants and young children who are at-risk for or have diagnosed disabilities. As readers will readily recognize, this is no small task: the "art" of effective intervention practices is continually subject to refinement and improvements of existing practices as well as introduction of entirely new ideas and approaches. As is the case with most topics subject to a rapid surge in scholarly attention, new findings and ideas are often steps ahead of their practical application and, in some cases, not easily translated into appropriate practices, creating what many have come to regard as a research-to-practice gap. Books in this series have been designed and prepared with an eye toward reducing this gap and assisting early childhood intervention personnel in becoming consumers of current theoretical and empirical information. The topics in the series are wide ranging and through explicit examples and discussion in each of the individual books offer a wealth of practical information to assist us all in providing the most effective interventions for families and their infants and young children.

The topic of the present volume is premature infants and their families, with a specific focus on the underlying rationale, design, and implementation of appropriate interventions. The general topic has received a great deal of attention in recent years and is reflected in a broad base of publications addressing varying aspects of the needs of premature babies and their families. What distinguishes this volume from others is the breadth of coverage with respect to critical practice issues. Dr. Wyly and her contributors have most effectively addressed the myriad of medical, educational, and environmental issues pertinent to the design and implementation of effective interventions for premature infants and their families. Further, they have managed to do such in a highly readable format that is packed with practical examples and practice exercises, not to mention the substantial reference lists for those wishing to gather additional information regarding a particular area. The result is a book that I would place on the "must read" list for an interdisciplinary audience including families, speech-language pathologists, psychologists, nurses, and other personnel who are involved in providing early intervention in hospital-based as well as community settings.

M. Jeanne Wilcox, Ph.D.
Series Editor

Preface

■

Change is a constant in the neonatal intensive care unit. From the era when many premature infants died and their parents were not allowed to visit their infants in the preterm nursery, there have been remarkable advances in neonatology. The technological advances have been continuous and have dramatically increased the survival rate of premature infants.

Professionals who care for these tiny newborns are now being challenged to look beyond the miraculous technological advances to include developmental and psychosocial components as part of their care. The medical model without appropriate developmental and psychosocial interventions for infants and their families is like the proverbial trying to clap with one hand.

This book addresses the developmental needs of preterm infants and psychosocial needs of families. The developmental needs of infants are seen within the framework of the medical care that must be delivered and the philosophy of family-centered neonatal care. Our goal is the stable development of the infant in the family, which is part of the infant's ongoing care from the time of birth.

One part of that goal is to provide a seamless system of early intervention referrals, which begin in the NICU and continue following discharge. For many high-risk infants, services that begin in the neonatal intensive care unit will continue long after discharge from the hospital. This will require making parents partners in the nonmedical care of their infants as well as ongoing collaboration of interdisciplinary teams with families.

Contributors

Jack Allen, M.A.
Curriculum Specialist
NICU Training Project
Buffalo State College
State University of New York
Buffalo, New York

Susan M. Pfalzer, R.N.C., M.S.
Clinical Nurse Specialist, NICU
Children's Hospital of Buffalo
Buffalo, New York

Mary R. Speth, R.N., B.S.N.
Project Coordinator
NICU Training Project
Buffalo State College
State University of New York
Buffalo, New York

Janet Rae Wilson, M.S., R.N., N.N.P.
Neonatal Outreach Coordinator
Children's Hospital of Buffalo
Buffalo, New York

M. Virginia Wyly, Ph.D.
Professor, Psychology
Buffalo State College
State University of New York
Buffalo, New York

Acknowledgments

■

We deeply appreciate the time and effort Mary Mueller spent typing this manuscript. Her good humor and attention to detail made our work much easier. We also appreciate the assistance of Robert Pollaro in preparing the references. Our gratitude to Richard C. Towne, Ph.D. for his skilled editorial guidance. Our special thanks to our NICU colleagues and to the families of premature infants who have guided us in understanding the wisdom of family-centered neonatal care.

Dedication

■

To Betty Dorr and Ann Bissonnette, friends who left us much too soon; also to Sarah Dorr Coppola our favorite premie, who is very much with us.

■ CHAPTER 1
Introduction

The history of man in the nine months
preceding his birth would probably be far
more interesting and attain events of
greater moment than all the three score and
ten year that follow it.
Samuel Taylor Coleridge

■ OVERVIEW

In the months prior to the birth of their baby, parents plan eagerly for the new arrival. But, parents-to-be usually do not plan for a premature birth. That is understandable, but at the same time, we should remember that approximately 7 to 9% of all births in the United States are premature, and nearly 4% are both premature and low birthweight (LBW). For example, in 1983, 9% of all births were less than 37 weeks gestation and over 6% of the babies weighed less than 2500 grams (5½ pounds) at birth (National Center for Health Statistics, 1985).

Such numbers are dramatic and demand attention. As a result, a growing body of literature that describes the relationship between prematurity and developmental outcomes has developed. The stresses of premature birth and deleterious perinatal events are major developmental risks for infants and young children. Not only are premature infants in jeopardy in early life, but their families experience difficulties as well. This chapter focuses on neonatal care for premature infants.

Our theme is developmental interventions for premature infants. We will review both historical and contemporary approaches to caring for preterm infants. Psychosocial interventions that can be used in Neonatal Intensive Care Units (NICU) to promote the well-being of infants and their families will be presented. The challenge of learning and collaborating across disciplines to provide support for the development of high-risk infants will be discussed. Other interventions for preterm infants and their families will be covered in subsequent chapters.

Your study of this text should enable you to:

- outline preterm infant development
- describe how preterm infant assessments are used to plan appropriate developmental interventions for preterm infants.
- outline current approaches to providing developmental interventions for fragile preterm infants both in the NICU and after discharge.
- describe family-centered neonatal care plans for preterm infants.

■ HOW TO USE THIS TEXT

You can do a number of things that will help you get the most out of this text.

- **Study with a purpose.** Approach each chapter with the chapter's general and specific outcomes in mind. Use the chapter outline to focus your attention on intended outcomes.
- **Review the highlighted terms.** Be sure you understand their meaning and how they are being used.
- **Use the case examples to clarify the content of the text.** Consider how they portray the content. Answer the questions about each study.

■ HISTORICAL PERSPECTIVE OF PRETERM CARE

Neonatology the study and treatment of newborns is relatively new. Although neonatology is generally acknowledged to have become firmly established over the past 30 years, the seeds of neonatology were planted in a hospital in Paris before the turn of the century.

In 1892 a French obstetrician, Pierre Budin, established a special unit in a Paris hospital for the care of sick and premature babies. He defined prematurity as newborn weight less than 2500 grams and published the first set of guidelines for the care of newborn infants. Budin's recommendations included maintaining temperature control and using gavage feeding to manage feeding problems (Budin, 1907). Budin's book contained a description of a device he and an associate, Etienne Stephene Tarnier, had designed for "weakling babies." It was the first incubator. Today, incubators and many of Budin's guidelines are still used in contemporary premature infant care.

Dr. Martin Couney, one of Budin's students, introduced Budin's techniques to the United States. Couney is best known for showing premature babies in incubators at World Fairs and other expositions throughout the United States and Europe. Dr. Couney called his incubators "child hatcheries" and demonstrated them initially at the

Berlin Exposition in 1896. For over 40 years Couney and his incubator road show astounded viewers who paid admission to see the miracle machines and the infants they kept alive (Liebling, 1939). The admission fee was waived for the parents who came to view their own infants. Couney's demonstrations influenced physicians in the United States to adopt the incubator and other innovative measures for preterm care.

In the United States, Dr. Julian Hess established the first premature infant unit in the 1920s at the Sarah Morris Hospital in Chicago. The unit used incubators and oxygen to increase the survival of "sickly" newborns. Hess and his associates also used feeding protocols based on the idea that neonatal mortality was related to overfeeding. In fact, the feeding schedule resulted in *underfeeding* premature babies (Hess & Lundeen, 1941). Much was still to be learned about newborn nutrition and their physiological problems.

Also during this period in the interest of regulating infection, hospital facilities began to restrict family visiting hours and to limit parent involvement in the care of their infant (Sammons & Lewis, 1985). From this start, the practice of limiting the parental role during an infant's hospitalization continued until the 1970s.

The medical care of premature infants changed very little between 1920 and 1940. During this period Ethel Dunham, director of the Division of Research in Child Development of the Children's Bureau in Washington, DC, collected data on premature infants. She published her findings in a book *Premature Infants: A Manual for Physicians* (Dunham, 1955). But the pace picked up a bit in the 1940s and 1950s. For example, researchers advanced our understanding of the diseases that affect preterm infants, and antibiotics were used increasingly to fight newborn infections.

During the 1960s major breakthroughs in medical knowledge and technology began to occur. New techniques were developed to assist preterm infants' breathing and to monitor their physiological functioning. Our understanding of diseases such as respiratory distress syndrome (RDS) and bronchopulmonary dysplasia (BPD) increased, and consequently the diseases were managed better. Research on pathology and on the growth and care of newborns focused attention on the special problems of preterm infants. At the same time, research findings began to change health care practices in the NICU.

New machinery and new types of health personnel found their way into the NICU. Regional perinatal centers were established throughout the United States and fragile newborn infants began to be transported from regional hospitals to new regional intensive care units. With these changes, the survival rate of premature and low birthweight infants has risen dramatically.

But as technology and health care personnel became more sophisticated, neonatal intensive care units became more impersonal. Neonatal intensive care units became busy places filled with machinery, and infants were cared for by many different, highly specialized medical staff. In the process, parents of the infants had little part in their infant's care. They sat in the waiting room, eclipsed by medical efforts to save the baby.

Other problems and ethical dilemmas have accompanied the remarkable advances in neonatal care. Today, surviving 1500 gram infants are commonplace, and many infants weighing 600 to 750 grams are routinely kept alive. Premature infants as young as 23 weeks gestation are surviving through the efforts of modern medicine.

With these changes, fundamental questions about the limits of medical efforts have arisen (Hack & Fanaroff, 1993; McCormick, 1994). Should heroic measures be taken to keep a 24-week baby alive when our most informed judgment says that child is likely to grow up with moderate to severe developmental disabilities? What are the probable developmental outcomes for very low birthweight and sick infants? What considerations should be given to the extraordinarily high cost of keeping sick premature infants alive?

By the mid 1980s NICU health providers began to acknowledge the need for enabling parents to fulfill their role as their infant's caregivers (Zeanah & Canger, 1983). NICU health providers recognized that the early parent-infant relationship that begins in the NICU is the groundwork for future interactions and for the infant's development. The move toward a family-centered focus in the NICU has gradually gained attention, but still is not universally accepted, and it is not always implemented (Ahmann, 1994; National Center for Family-Centered Care, 1990). For the most part intensive care nurseries are still infant-centered, not family-centered, in their philosophy and approach. Currently NICU staff are challenged to find ways to promote supportive interactions between parents and infants. If there are to be positive long-term outcomes, such psychosocial interventions need to be in place both in the NICU and at home (or in other discharge settings).

■ NEONATAL CARE FOR PRETERM INFANTS

The **neonatal** period is the first 30 days of life. During this period newly born infants are known as newborns. The first 48 hours after being born is the time when newborns are most likely to die, and the following first weeks of life can be critical to preterm infants' survival and development.

Care for premature infants is not new; they have always required special care in order to survive. Some of the more famous survivors include Mark Twain, Albert Einstein, Isaac Newton, Winston Churchill, the Dionne quintuplets, and Charles Darwin. Today, attitudes on how to care for preterm infants are influenced in part by the early efforts to care for babies born "too soon." Now, let us turn to some current concerns in caring for newly born preterm infants.

Neonatal Intensive Care

In the United States, intensive care is provided for approximately 250,000 newborns each year (Gottfried, 1985). The average hospital stay for premature infants is 15 days, but some infants may be hospitalized for weeks or even months (Gottfried, Hodgman, & Brown, 1985). The specialized care for sick newborns is costly (see Figure 1–1). Hospitalization costs generally exceed $500 per day (Ensher & Clark, 1994).

There are three levels of neonatal intensive care in the United States. The level designation assigned to a neonatal unit indicates the extent of care available. The care level of a neonatal patient facility depends on the needs, resources, and geographical location of an area. A Level One facility is a hospital that cares for mothers and infants with no risk factors. Management of normal pregnancies and births is Level One's primary function. If a problem arises, these hos-

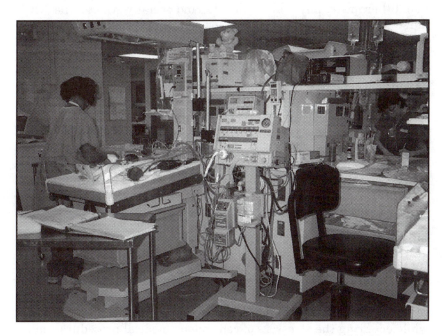

Figure 1–1. Neonatal Intensive Care Unit. (Photograph courtesy of Children's Hospital of Buffalo Department of Medical Photography.)

pitals have support equipment available for the infant until transport to a higher level facility takes place.

A Level Two unit provides services for mothers and infants who require intensive care treatment. But specialized services such as neurosurgery and cardiac surgery are often unavailable in these hospitals. Often, infants in Level Three units are back transferred to less intensive Level Two once they are stable but still need care. Level Two units are usually located in both urban and suburban areas.

A Level Three facility is equipped to handle the medical problems of very ill newborns and their mothers (see Figure 1–1). Many Level Three units are regional perinatal centers that provide outreach services and education for other units. A complete range of neonatal and pediatric medical care is provided in these units. Very early premature infants, sick newborns, and infants with respiratory and cardiac problems are cared for in Level Three units. Transport of infants from Level One and Level Two facilities and from outlying areas is usually part of Level Three services.

Multidisciplinary Teams

Care for high-risk infants and their families in the NICU is done by multidisciplinary teams. The team consists of physicians, neonatal nurses, respiratory therapists, speech-language pathologists, occupational therapists, physical therapists, and social workers. The NICU nurse has primary responsibility for continuity of the infant's care, with consultation with other professionals on the NICU team. Recently, some NICUs have added infant specialists, psychologists, and parent advocates to their staff. These professionals support staff to provide developmental care and family interventions.

With the passage of Public Law 99-457, the hospital has been idenified as a site for early intervention for infants with disabilities and their families. These early intervention services must be provided by professionals from several disciplines who work together to assist infants and their families. More NICUs are now incoporating early interventionists into their professional staff. These professionals plan early intervention in the NICU and assist transition for infants and their families to community-based intervention programs.

NICU Environment

Infants begin life in the womb, a warm, well-modulated nurturing environment. Infants born prematurely, however, unexpectedly enter what is often a noisy, brightly lit, and impersonal intensive care environment. Preterm infants attempt to cope with this environment while enduring the stressors of continuous medical procedures, many of them painful. Because of their immaturity premature infants are easily taxed by the excessive stimulation that is typical of care in neonatal intensive care units (VandenBerg, 1985).

The neonatal intensive care unit (NICU) evolved over the past 20 years to provide needed medical and life support for premature infants, low birthweight infants, and infants with medical problems. A walk through a NICU reveals a busy, noisy environment dominated by machinery. Indeed, the overwhelming array of equipment is a primary characteristic of NICUs. The medical staff are highly specialized and trained to respond to the ever present potential for a crisis.

It has been suggested that the extrauterine experience has potentially adverse developmental consequences for premature infants (Gottfried, 1985). Although most follow-up developmental studies show that preterm infants develop normally, there is increasing evidence of cognitive and sensory defects among very low birthweight babies (Blackburn, 1995; Blackburn & Barnard, 1985; Saigal, Szatmari, Rosenbaum, Campbell, & King, 1991).

As a consequence, questions are being raised about the quality of the intensive care environment and its impact on fragile premature infants. Adapting the NICU environment to meet the needs of fragile infants has become a concern for health professionals.

Developmental Care Procedures

In modern neonatal intensive care units a variety of developmental caregiving procedures have been initiated to help modify the infant's environment and to help the infant cope with excessive stimulation. A premature infant's immature central nervous system can result in behavioral disorganization and poor regulation of sleep and alert states. These difficulties are compounded by medical and caregiving procedures which in the NICU are sometimes done without considering the infant's behavioral state of consciousness or stress level.

Optimal developmental care has been designed and implemented to minimize infant stress and outcomes (Als et al., 1988; Lefrak-Okikawa & Lund, 1993). Developmental care includes reducing excessive noise and light levels in the NICU, utilizing day/night lighting patterns, proper positioning and handling, and individualizing care procedures.

Currently, controlled studies are being done to assess the impact of developmental care on infant outcomes. Initial results show that developmental care protocols reduce the average hospital stay in the Level Three NICU (Als et al., 1986). Als and colleagues have found that developmental intervention in the NICU resulted in a number of positive outcomes including shorter hospital stay, shorter time on the ventilator, and fewer medical complications.

Developmental care is being incorporated into routine care practices in the NICU. It is designed to minimize infant stress, facilitate self-organization, and promote infant stability and recovery.

Parent Experience With Preterm Infant

Given the condition of their baby, it is not surprising that preterm infants' families experience difficulties as well. Feelings of inadequacy, anger, and grief are often a part of the family experience in the NICU. Parents may experience anxiety over the fragile state of their infant. "Will my baby live or die?" is a commonly asked question.

The baby's medical condition is not the only source of such concerns. Because of their poor motor stability and difficulty maintaining alertness, preterm infants do not engage in the social interactions typical of term infants. Preterm infants' cues and interaction signals are often weak and disorganized and too often missed. Typically, parents do not understand what is happening and they begin to feel incompetent as caregivers. Simply put, parents often lack the resources needed to cope with the demands of their vulnerable infants. Consequently, the support of NICU health professionals is essential for families as well as for preterm infants.

Practices in the NICU are changing to provide formal and informal family support (Consolvo, 1987). Families are being encouraged to take a more active role in the nonmedical care of their infant (Plaas, 1994).

■ DEVELOPMENTAL OUTCOMES

The past decade has been characterized by increasing concern for the developmental and psychological outcomes of high-risk infants who begin their lives in a neonatal intensive care nursery (Gorski, 1986; Schwartz, 1981). Statistics show that high-risk neonates are at risk for developmental deficiencies, motor handicaps and cognitive and sensory deficits, and infant abuse and neglect (Levene & Dubowitz, 1982; Meisels, Plunkett, Roloff, Pasick, & Stiefel, 1986). There is growing evidence that serious developmental problems are most likely to occur in the population of very early and very low birthweight infants. This group includes 10–15% of all fragile infants. In addition, approximately 15% of preterm and low birthweight infants suffer moderate disabilities such as learning problems. The remaining population, approximately 70%, have mild developmental problems such as learning disorders, motor deficits, and attention deficits or they develop normally (Cohen, 1987; Goldberg & DiVitto, 1983).

Although the developmental progress for infants in the NICU is encouraging, questions are being raised about the long-term developmental outcome of medically fragile infants who are being kept alive as a result of technological advances. These infants often endure biological, environmental, and medical insults associated with aggressive medical treatments and long hospitalizations.

What are the long-term effects of these practices on infant development? As sicker populations of very low birthweight and preterm infants survive, there is a concern that these infants will show severe resultant developmental problems and disabilities. Unfortunately these concerns still cannot be addressed until a well developed, generally accepted body of data about outcomes is available. We need longitudinal studies of the developmental status of infants who have been hospitalized. Questions need to be answered regarding the effects of the NICU environment as well as medical care practice. Such studies will provide data and information. Answers will come from interpretation of this data.

■ DEFINING AND EXPLAINING PREMATURITY

Before the 1960s, infants were classified as premature according to their weight. Infants who weighed less than 2500 grams (5½ pounds) at birth were designated premature. Infants who weighed more than 2500 grams at birth were identified as full term. These definitions proved inadequate, however, since the duration of gestation was not used to determine newborn maturity.

In 1961, the World Health Organization identified the term *low birthweight* as a designation for newborn infants weighing less than 2500 grams. This definition also disregarded gestation age. More recently, however, the World Health Organization developed new criteria that resulted in the following designations:

Full-term	Infants born between 37 to 42 weeks gestation.
Premature	Infants born prior to 37 weeks gestation.
Postterm	Infants born after 42 weeks gestation.
Small for Gestational Age (SGA)	Infants born at or after 37 weeks gestation and who are underweight for gestational age.
Small-for-Date and Premature	Infants with slow interuterine growth born prior to 37 weeks.

Appropriate Growth for Gestational Age (AGA)	Infants with normal interuterine growth at the time of birth. They are small, however, because they are premature.
Low Birthweight	Less than 2500 grams (LBW)
Very Low Birthweight	Less than 1500 grams (VBLW)

Consider the following examples:

Infant Alex was born at 37 weeks and weighed 2400 grams.

Catlin was born at 35 weeks and weighed 2800 grams.

Prior to 1960, Alex but not Catlin would be classified as premature. Current definitions, however, would classify Alex as full term, SGA and Catlin as premature.

Gestational age is estimated in several ways. One common technique is to count the number of weeks since the last day of the last menstrual period. This method may result in miscalculation when the mother's recollection is faulty or if there have been irregular menses. During the prenatal period, estimates of fetal age are obtained from physical milestones of the developing fetus such as fundal height (height of the uterine fundus above the symphysis pubis). After birth, gestational age is often determined by physical examination of the newborn that includes assessment of neurologic responses.

Studies have documented that the youngest and smallest infants are at greatest risk for infant mortality and morbidity. Infants considered to be at the most risk of complications and death are those under 1000 grams or less than 32 weeks gestational age.

■ EPIDEMIOLOGY AND PREMATURITY RISK

Epidemiology

This section focuses on the epidemiology of prematurity in the United States as well as related causative indicators of prematurity. While epidemiological patterns of premature births provide clues to causation, the actual causes of prematurity are still unknown.

The incidence of prematurity is associated with socioeconomic factors (Kotelchuck & Wise, 1987). While premature births occur in all economic classes, women of lower socioeconomic status (SES) are more likely to have premature births. There are several explanations for this. Poor women often have little access to good prenatal care, and their nutrition and living conditions are often inadequate. Moreover, more teenage pregnancies occur among low SES groups, and teenage mothers are at risk for low birthweight births (Institute of Medicine, 1985). The effects of poverty on prematurity points up the need to provide prenatal and postnatal care for mothers of infants across SES groups.

In the United States, socioeconomic status and race are related so it is no surprise that prematurity is also associated with race. In fact, the prematurity rate for blacks is more than two times that of whites. Although black births are only 16% of all births nationwide, 29% of all premature infants are born to black women (National Center for Health Statistics, 1985). Similarly, low birthweight is greater among blacks than among whites. During the 1970s and 1980s the overall rate of LBW and prematurity declined more among whites than among blacks.

The geographical distribution of prematurity and low birthweight reflects the distribution of the poor and minorities who lack preventive health services. Thus, across the United States the rates of prematurity and LBW vary from state to state and within regions depending on where the poor populations reside. Where there are many poor people and minorities there will be more premature infants and LBW babies, and where there are few poor people and minorities there will be fewer premature infants and LBW babies. It is misleading, however, to assume that prematurity is simply an outcome of poverty. Approximately half of the premature births are not associated with the risk factors of poverty or age.

Prematurity Risk

Although specific factors that cause prematurity and low birthweight have not been pinpointed, there are a number of maternal risk factors associated with poor birth outcomes (Creasy, Gummer, & Liggins, 1980; Giblin, Poland, Waller, & Ager, 1988). Some maternal risk factors associated with prematurity and low birthweight are multiple pregnancy, maternal infections during pregnancy, poor obstetric history, genetic factors, substance abuse, smoking, and poor nutrition.

A maternal history of previous birth problems is the single strongest predictor of subsequent premature birth. This is not surprising because mothers who live in poor, crowded conditions, lack prenatal care, and have inadequate nutrition are more likely to have health problems that affect the developing fetus.

Maternal health problems during the prenatal period are also a strong predictor of prematurity. Mothers with chronic illnesses such as high blood pressure or heart disease are more likely to deliver early. Multiple pregnancy also contributes to a shortened pregnancy.

When more than one fetus is being supported by the reproductive system, adequate growth is less likely to occur, consequently multiple births are often associated with low birthweight and premature.

Finally, prematurity is more likely to occur when the mother's reproductive system is immature. Thus, young adolescent mothers are more likely to have premature babies.

The question of why a baby is born prematurely is still unanswered. Evidence suggests that women from disadvantaged socioeconomic conditions are at risk for premature and LBW births because of the many adverse factors associated with poverty. Yet approximately 50% of premature births are seemingly unexplained. These babies are born of healthy parents with adequate resources, good health care, and no previous history of birth problems. The fact that there is no adequate explanation of the cause of prematurity can exacerbate the anxiety that parents experience in NICUs.

■ SUMMARY

Each year approximately 250,000 of the babies born in the United States are placed in neonatal intensive care units. There is a growing body of evidence that developmental problems may arise in very small, medically fragile premature infants.

Although the services provided in NICUs reflect remarkable technological and medical advances, there is considerable evidence that the NICU environment can tax premature infants. Lifesaving medical procedures, although necessary, may also stress premature infants. NICU health professionals are exploring ways to address this problem by employing developmental care practices to reduce infants' stress and to optimize their development through behavioral and environmental interventions.

Neonatology, the study and treatment of newborn infants, is a relatively recent phenomenon in the United States. Care for premature infants takes place in neonatal intensive care units. There are three levels of intensive care treatment facilities for high-risk infants in the United States. NICU levels are determined by the infant populations they serve. The Level One unit is for no or low risk premature deliveries, the Level Two unit is for intensive care, while Level Three units serve fragile premature infants. Current care reflects the remarkable technological and medical advances made in the field over the past 20 years. Care is primarily infant-centered; family care is only just beginning.

Epidemiological studies of prematurity show that both premature and low birthweight births are associated with socioeconomic status and race. Poor prenatal health care, maternal illness, and prior birth difficulties are strong predictive factors for prematurity. However, approximately 50% of all premature births are not characterized by such conditions. In fact, we are still uncertain about the causes of premature births.

REFERENCES

Ahmann, E. (1994). Family-centered care: Shifting orientation. *Pediatric Nursing, 20*, 113–117.

Als, H., Lawhon, G., Brown, E., Gibes, R., Duffy, F. H., McAnulty, G., & Blickman, J. (1986). Individualized behavioral and environmental care for the very low birth weight preterm infant at risk for bronchopulmonary dysplasia: Neonatal intensive care unit and developmental outcomes. *Pediatrics, 78*, 1123–1132.

Als, H., Lawhon, G., Gibes, R., Duffy, F. H., McAnulty, G. R., & Blickman, J. G. (1988, February). *Individualized behavioral and environmental care for the very low birth weight preterm infant at high risk for bronchopulomonary dysplasia and intraventricular hemorrhage. Study II: NICU outcome.* Paper presented at the Annual Meeting of the New England Perinatal Society, Woodstock, VT.

Blackburn, S. (1995). Problems of preterm infants after discharge. *Journal of Obstetric, Gynecologic and Neonatal Nursing, 24*, 43–49.

Blackburn, S., & Barnard, K. E. (1985). Analysis of caregiving events relating to preterm infants in the special care unit. In A. W. Gottfried & J. L. Gaiter (Eds.), *Infant stress under intensive care* (pp. 113–129). Baltimore: University Park Press.

Budin, P. (1907). *The nursling.* London: Caxton.

Cohen, S. E. (1987). Longitudinal studies of preterm infants. In H. W. Taeusch & M. W. Yogman (Eds.), *Follow-up management of the high-risk infant* (pp. 21–28). Boston, MA: Little, Brown and Company.

Consolvo, C. A. (1987). Siblings in the NICU. *Neonatal Network, 5*, 7–11.

Creasy, R., Gummer, B., & Liggins, G. (1980). System for predicting spontaneous preterm birth. *Obstetrics and Gynecology, 55*, 692–695.

Dunham, E. (1955). *Premature infants: A manual for physicians* (2nd ed.). New York: Paul B. Hoeber.

Ensher, G. L., & Clark, D. A. (1994). *Newborns at risk.* Gaithersburg, MD: Aspen.

Giblin, P. T., Poland, M. C., Waller, J. B., & Ager, J.W. (1988). Correlates of neonatal morbidity: Maternal characteristics and family resources. *Journal of Genetic Psychology, 149*, 527–533.

Goldberg, S., & DiVitto, B. A. (1983). *Born too soon.* San Francisco, CA: W. H. Freeman.

Gorski, P. (1986, October). *Neurodevelopmental risks and the politics of change.* Paper presented at Developmental Interventions in Neonatal Care Conference, Chicago, IL.

Gottfried, A. (1985). Environment of newborn infants in special care units. In A. W. Gottfried & J. L. Gaiter (Eds.), *Infant stress under intensive care* (pp. 23–54). Baltimore: University Park Press.

Gottfried, A. W., Hodgman, J. E., & Brown, K. W. (1985, June). *How intensive is newborn intensive care? An environmental analysis.* Paper presented at Developmental Interventions in Neonatal Care Conference, Washington, DC.

Hack, M., & Fanaroff, A. A. (1993). Outcomes of extremely immature infants—A perinatal dilemma. *The New England Journal of Medicine, 329,* 1649–1650.

Hess, J. H., & Lundeen, E. C. (1941). *The premature infant.* Philadelphia: Lippincott.

Institute of Medicine. (1985). *Preventing low birth weight.* Washington, DC: National Academy Press.

Kotelchuck, M. C., & Wise, P. H. (1987). Epidemiology of prematurity and goals for prevention. In H. W. Taeusch & M. W. Yogman (Eds.), *Follow-up management of the high-risk infant* (pp. 3–14). Boston, MA: Little, Brown and Company.

Lefrak-Okikawa, L., & Lund, C. H. (1993). Nursing practices in the neonatal intensive care unit. In M. H. Klaus & A. A. Fanaroff (Eds.), *Care of the high-risk neonate* (pp. 212–227). Philadelphia: W. B. Saunders.

Levene, M., & Dubowitz, L. (1982) Low birthweight babies: Long term follow-up. *British Journal of Hospital Medicine, 37,* 158–165.

Liebling, A. J. (1939, Summer). Patron of the premies. *Readers Digest,* 20–24.

McCormick, M. C. (1994). Survival of very tiny babies—Good news and bad news. *The New England Journal of Medicine, 331,* 802–803.

Meisels, S. J., Plunkett, J. W., Roloff, D. W., Pasick, P. L., & Stiefel, G. S. (1986). Growth and development of preterm infants with respiratory distress syndrome and bronchopulmonary dysplasia. *Pediatrics, 77,* 345–352.

National Center for Health Statistics. (1985). *Advanced report of final natality statistics.* Monthly Vital Statistics Report Series, *34*(6), [Suppl.] (publication No. PHS 85-1120). Hyattsville, MD: U.S. Department of Health and Human Services.

National Center for Family-Centered Care. (1990). *What is family-centered care?* Bethesda, MD: Association for the Care of Children's Health.

Plaas, K. M. (1994). The evolution of parental roles in the NICU. *Neonatal Nursing, 6,* 31–33.

Saigal, S., Szatmari, P., Rosenbaum, P., Campbell, D., & King, S. (1991). Cognitive abilities and school performance of extremely low birth weight children and matched term control children at age 8 years: A regional study. *Journal of Pediatrics, 118,* 757–760.

Sammons, A. H., & Lewis, M. (1985) *Premature babies: A different beginning.* St. Louis: C. V. Mosby.

Schwartz, D. (1981). Intensive care nurseries: Making them more human. *Children Today,* 41–42.

VandenBerg, K. (1985). Revising the traditional model: An individualized approach to developmental interventions in the intensive care nursery. *Neonatal Network, 3,* 32–38.

Zeanah, C. H., & Canger, C. I. (1983). The mental health professional in the intensive care nursery. *Zero to Three, 4,* 1–6.

■ CHAPTER 2

Behavior and Development
of the Preterm Infant

Learn of the Muse, and may thy
Pains succeed, Don't, 'till 'tis born,
defer thy Pions care; Begin betime,
and for its Birth prepare.
Paedotrophia, Scevole De St. Marthe,
1579

■ INTRODUCTION

Being born too soon means that neonates must adapt to life outside the womb, although they are neurologically and physiologically unprepared for the demands of the undertaking. It is often a very difficult process.

Premature and low birthweight infants experience a significantly greater number of problems during labor and the birth process than do full-term infants placing them at risk for subsequent developmental problems (Kitchen & Murton, 1985). Batshaw and Perrelt (1986) state that the youngest and smallest infants are at a disadvantage of getting a good start on survival and adaptation to the extrauterine world. Because of the immaturity of their body organs, they may not have the normal functioning typical of full-term infants. They are more likely to have breathing difficulties because of their less mature lungs, and they are more likely to have jaundice and difficulty maintaining temperature control. Their growth potential may be restricted. There is a higher probability of brain damage among this population because of physiological or metabolic events. Neonatal mortality increases with infants' decreased gestational age and birthweight.

While starting at an earlier gatepost than do their full-term peers, and often with a risky physiological status, premature infants' developmental progress also depends on their medical interventions and on their response to the overwhelming NICU environment. Understanding these influences on premature infants' development and behavior can help parents, who are parents "too soon," cope better with the unexpected birth of their infant.

Knowledge and recognition of changes in the developmental status of high-risk infants in the NICU serve as the basis for assessment and subsequent intervention. Further, understanding the organization of neurologic functioning during this period in the face of various environmental events is useful in anticipating later neuromotor outcomes. There are, for example, numerous studies of the deleterious relationship of interventricular hemorrhages, bleeding in the brain ventricles, to later cognitive functioning (Als, 1986; Narayan, 1986).

In this chapter we will look at neonatal consequences of premature labor and delivery and common medical problems associated with prematurity. We will examine the development and behavior of premature infants. Premature infants' behavioral organization and control of the sleep-wake cycle will be described. Change in patterns of neurological functioning in premature infants will be highlighted.

■ CONSEQUENCES OF PREMATURE LABOR AND BIRTH

I was in my seventh month of pregnancy. My husband and I were anticipating our first born. We had started LaMaze classes and shopped for baby furniture. My office staff had a surprise baby shower for me. I would describe that period as one of the happiest times in my life. I was simply unprepared for what happened next. Early one morning I woke up with severe stomach cramps, at least that's what I thought it was. After several hours, my husband called our physician who told us to meet her at the hospital as quickly as possible.

There was no waiting at the hospital; an emergency medical team began to monitor me immediately. My physician told me that all indications were that I would deliver but reassured me that they were ready to meet any complications that might arise. I was so frightened. I delivered a baby boy a few hours later. I saw him only briefly because he was taken to the intensive care nursery. He had difficulty breathing and was so very small.

It's difficult to describe the enormous let down I felt. Somehow I felt like a failure. It was even more difficult because I was in the hospital and didn't see my baby for several days. My husband had the burden of talking to doctors, telling friends and family and comforting me. Actually, we both needed comforting. Fortunately, the story has a happy ending. After three weeks my baby came home and a year later is doing fine. Still, I remember that experience with sadness and wonder why it happened.

This case illustrates that a premature birth experience is difficult not only for the baby but also for the parents. Like the baby, the parents are unprepared for the abrupt delivery. Their baby is not what they expected; it is small and fragile. They are often fearful about the baby's medical condition and feel guilty and out of control. The emotional roller coaster so often described by parents of premature infants will be explored more fully in Chapters 8 and 9. In this section, some causes of premature labor and delivery and the consequences of a premature birth will be examined.

Labor

Labor is the process by which the fetus descends from the uterus and is expelled from the birth canal. Labor begins when the contractions occur at regular intervals (Creasy & Resnick, 1989). Labor actually consists of uterine contractions which provide the force needed to propel the fetus downward. The exact trigger for labor is not known. Researchers have identified an increase in the concentration of the hormone prostaglandin in the amniotic fluid and blood. This may influence the onset of uterine contractions (Karim, 1968).

Other investigators have shown that progesterone concentrations diminish at the onset of labor (Kumar, Goodno, & Barnes, 1962). Researchers speculate that the hormone progesterone, when present in large amounts, relaxes the muscles of the uterus, which in turn depresses uterine contractility. However, recent studies have confirmed that progesterone does not decrease toward the end of pregnancy but rather there is an increase in the receptor sites for two other hormones, estrogen and oxytocin, the smooth muscle cells of the uterus, the myometrium. The production of these receptor sites in the uterus is now thought to be the mechanism responsible for the onset of labor (Challis & Mitchell, 1981; Wallenburg, 1983).

Uterine contractions bring about the dilation and effacement of the cervix. The contractions also propel the descent of the fetus in preparation for the birth process.

The term **labor** describes the muscular work that must be done to propel the infant through the birth canal. Some mothers experience 2 days of labor, whereas others experience only a few hours.

Normal labor proceeds in three stages:

Stage One: In this stage cervical dilation begins. The stage ends when cervical dilation and effacement are completed, that is, when the cervix is dilated to 10 centimeters. This is the longest phase of labor and lasts on the average 6.5 hours. For first-time pregnancies, this phase is typically longer, that is, approximately 8 to 14 hours.

Stage Two: This stage begins with the start of the expulsion of the fetus. The regular contractions push the baby through the vagina. It ends with the birth of the baby. Typically this stage lasts for 1 to 2 hours.

Stage Three: This phase is marked by the expulsion of the placenta or afterbirth. This stage lasts from 15 minutes to 1 hour.

Why a woman goes into premature labor is still unknown. There are many maternal factors associated with premature birth. For example, women who carry twins are more likely to deliver prematurely. Early rupture of the placenta (abruptio placentae) stimulates early onset of labor, fetal hemorrhage, and neonatal shock at birth.

Teenage mothers, low income mothers, and mothers with poor health histories are at increased risk for prematurity. Other factors associated with prematurity risk include poor prenatal care, smoking and drug use during pregnancy, kidney infection, toxemia, and multiple or closely spaced pregnancies.

Low birthweight infant births are also associated with a number of material and environmental factors. Drug use, for example, heroin, cocaine, nicotine, and alcohol, is related to low birthweight. Lack of prenatal care and poor nutrition are also tied to low birthweight. Yet, no single cause has been positively identified. Uncertainty about the cause of prematurity may result in feelings of frustration and guilt between parents whose infant has been born prematurely.

Currently, sophisticated medical procedures are available to detect potential problems with the fetus and to ascertain labor and birth difficulties that might jeopardize the newborn (Babson, Benson, Pernoll, & Benda, 1980). Careful monitoring of the fetus can assess fetal well-being. Fetal monitoring is used when the baby is thought to be at risk for serious complications during labor and delivery.

Fetal **monitoring** involves using several procedures to evaluate the fetus throughout pregnancy. An ultrasound monitor is used to estimate fetal growth, activity, respiration, movements, and the amount of amniotic fluid (Philip, 1987). External monitors are used to measure patterns of fetal heart rate. Abnormalities in fetal heart rate, **tachycardia** (rapid heart rate) or **bradycardia** (low heart rate), can be detected through fetal monitoring, and interventions can be implemented if needed. During labor, measurement of fetal PH may be done using intermittent scalp blood samples. This indicates whether the fetus is compensating metabolically for the stress associated with labor. Fetal monitoring can provide indications of distress such as loss of oxygen, sudden change in fetal respiration or heart rate that can cause brain damage, perinatal cardiac and respiratory difficulties, or even death. These techniques provide guidelines for physicians in their management of fetal development and delivery.

Effect of Labor and Delivery on the Fetus

Labor is hard on any fetus. It requires tremendous adaptation to the rapid changes that precede neonatal life. Stresses occur, for example, when the uterine contractions decrease placental perfusion, which in turn creates an oxygen deficit for the fetus. Oxygen levels are restored each time the uterus relaxes. Another stress results from increased interuterine pressure caused by the uterus contracting in the absence of the cushion of amniotic fluid which has been lost due to the rupture of the membranes. A specific example deals with pressure on the infant's head. Normally in preparation for delivery, the fetus moves so that the head is downward. As the fetus descends from the uterus, it is propelled by uterine contractions which, depending on their intensity, can result in intercranial hemorrhages.

Obviously, the birth process is traumatic for all babies. As babies exit through the narrow birth canal there is pressure on the head causing head molding. This is usually present in some degree in all vertex births. Bruises to the face and skull are common as are cephalhematomas caused by bleeding under the skin surface as the skin rubs against the pelvic bones. Despite the stress of birth, most infants recover and adapt to their extrauterine existence without long-term deleterious effects.

But when labor is difficult or abnormal, such as during a breech (feet first) presentation or face and shoulder presentation, there is an increase in perinatal mortality and morbidity. **Fetal distress** occurs when there is a rapid change in heart pattern or decrease in oxygen. With difficult labor and delivery, there is a greater risk of fetal brain damage or loss of oxygen. Injuries to the head can cause excessive pressure and bleeding inside the scalp, termed **intraventricular hemorrhage**. When fetal distress is suspected, fetal monitoring is done during labor and childbirth.

Premature labor often occurs when there is placental abruptio or a premature separation of a normally implanted placenta. This premature separation results in asphyxia and may produce neonatal shock during or immediately after birth.

At birth, newborn status is usually determined using the Apgar scoring system (Apgar, 1953) which evaluates five signs of a newborn's condition at 1 and 5 minutes after birth. The conditions include: respiration, heart rate, muscle tone, irritability, and color. Each component is scored from 0 to 2, with the total maximum score of 10. A total score of 0 to 3 indicates severe distress, 4 to 6 represents some difficulty, and 7 to 10 signifies little or no distress. Table 2–1 shows the Apgar scoring system.

Infants born prematurely, because of the extreme urgency of their medical condition may not be assessed using an Apgar rating.

TABLE 2–1. Apgar Scale

Function	0	1	2
Heart Rate	No Heartbeat	Blow 100	100–140 beats per minute
Muscle Tone	Limp muscle tone	Moderate	Flexed extremities Good muscle tone
Respiratory	No breathing	Irregular breathing Weak cry	Regular breathing Strong cry
Reflex Response to Stimulation	No response	Slow response	Facial grimace Cough or sneeze
Color	Blue or grey	Pink body but blue extremities	Body completely pink

Instead, procedures are quickly put into place to stabilize them immediately and to prevent further problems that can lead to central nervous system damage and physiological dysfunction. At birth, newborns lose heat rapidly but quickly begin to regulate their temperature. Low birthweight and premature infants have more difficulty managing their body temperature. Consequently, they are often placed on radiant warmers to provide heat. Heart rate and breathing are then assessed. Thermal regulation must begin immediately because of the rapid heat loss that occurs at the time of birth.

If an infant's respiration is compromised, oxygen may be administered through manual ventilation, which is bag and mask placed over the infant's face. The bag ventilation provides 100% oxygen. In the event that manual ventilation is unsuccessful, intubation and ventilation via the trachea may be used. This procedure involves inserting an endotracheal tube with bag to tube ventilator using 100% oxygen. Cardiac stimulants or massage may be given to newborns with cardiovascular difficulties. High-risk newborns experience a number of problems that must be anticipated and treated as part of routine care.

■ COMMON PROBLEMS IN PRETERM INFANTS

Many problems that occur among premature and low birthweight infants can jeopardize the infant's immediate well being or have an impact on long-term development. Several critical problems commonly observed among preterm infants will be outlined in this section. For a more in-depth discussion of medical problems associated with prematurity, the reader is referred to *Care of the High-Risk Neonate* (Klaus & Fanaroff, 1993).

Respiratory Disorders

Because preterm infants are born with immature lungs, many respiratory diseases characterize the neonatal period. In fact the most frequent causes of neonatal morbidity and mortality are respiratory disorders (Korones, 1986).

The development of the fetal lungs takes place over three phases (Daze', 1985). The *glandular* phase takes place in the first 4 months. In this period the two primary bronchial branches appear, followed by the branching of the bronchi which is completed by 16 weeks. The next phase is the *canalicular phase* which continues to 24 weeks. This phase is marked by a proliferation of vascular and capillary networks and the formation of respiratory bronchiolus. Terminal air sacs appear. By 24 weeks respiration outside the uterus can be supported by ventilators in some infants. The *alveolar* phase is the final period of lung development. In this phase the true air pockets (alveolar) clusters mature and capillaries proliferate. By 37 weeks enough of the substance known as surfactant, a substance that coats the alveoli of the lungs and prevents them from collapsing, is produced for respiratory stability.

Surfactant is a complex lipoprotein that binds to the lung's surface and reduces surface tension wherever there is interplay between the air and water. The presence of surfactant lowers the pressure that can cause collapse of the alveoli. By 37 weeks the presence of thin-walled alveoli and ongoing surfactant production allows newborn infants to breathe independently.

Several types of respiratory problems will be examined in this section. At least 50% of premature infants experience some signs and symptoms of respiration distress. The severity of outcome of respiratory distress depends on the infant's age and the type of intervention used.

Respiratory Distress Syndrome

Respiratory distress syndrome (RDS), also known as hyalin membrane disease, one of the most common problems in premature infants, affects between 10 to 20% of preterm infants. The percentage affected rises to 65% in infants weighing less than 1000 grams. The incidence of RDS increases the earlier the birth. RDS accounts for 15 to 20% of neonatal mortality (Perelman & Farrell, 1982).

Lung maturity and sufficient lung surfactant are necessary for normal, functional respiration. Respiratory distress syndrome occurs because of immature lung development accompanied by surfactant deficiency. At birth the first breaths taken by an infant dispel the fluid in the lungs and stabilize the alveoli. Premature infants with RDS appear to breathe normally after birth due to residual surfactant on the alveoli walls. However, as the surfactant becomes dissipated, breathing becomes labored and the alveoli collapse. Subsequent breaths require tremendous effort as the infant tries to inflate the alveoli. As the infant attempts to increase breathing efforts, grunting, nasal flaring and synchrony in breathing is evident. Early in RDS, hypoxia develops resulting in respiratory acidosis (high carbon dioxide levels) and alveolar necrosis (lesion of alveoli).

Clinical management of RDS involves identifying infants at risk for RDS through monitoring skin color, blood gases, temperature, and heart rate. Mechanical ventilation or other ventilatory support is used to alleviate pulmonary disfunction. Mechanical ventilation allows an exchange of oxygen and carbon dioxide. Surfactant treatment using exogenous surfactant preparations is currently used as an RDS management therapy (Merritt & Hallman, 1988). Infants with surfactant deficiency are candidates for surfactant replacement therapy. Two surfactant products are currently being used in the United States, Esosurf Neonatal™ and Survanta™ (Shapiro, 1992). For most infants, treatment combined with developing lung maturity, usually results in gradual recovery.

Apnea

Apnea is defined as the cessation of breathing for longer than 15 seconds. Breathing in premature infants is irregular and interspersed with pauses. When the pause is longer than 15 seconds it is known as an apneic episode. Of the many factors related to apnea in premature infants, the most common is immaturity of the central nervous system respiratory centers. Medullary respiratory regulator centers are immature and have depressed functioning in very premature infants. Consequently, apnea is likely to occur. Left undetected or untreated, apnea can result in hypoxemic damage or even death.

Interventions such as ventilation, bag and mask resuscitation, and rocking water beds have been used to correct the problem. Apnea monitors, which signal an alarm when the infant stops breathing, are used in hospitals and at home after discharge. Regular respiration increases and apnea decreases with maturation of the central nervous system.

Asphyxia

Asphyxia is a dysfunction in the exchange of oxygen and carbon dioxide, which results in hypoxia or decreased levels of oxygen and diminished cerebral blood flow. The human brain is dependent on continuous cerebral blood perfusion. When the cerebral blood flow is lowered, the self-regulation of the brain's blood supply is impaired, which in turn leads to brain swelling and hemorrhage. Thus, asphyxia is the primary cause of central nervous system (CNS) damage before and after birth.

Neonatal care of asphyxiated infants involves a number of procedures, all of which depend on accurate assessment of the infant's condition and responsiveness. Resuscitation techniques that establish good ventilation and adequate oxygenation levels are most commonly employed. Fluid balance, cardiac massage, and maintenance of normal blood pressure are also used in resuscitation approaches. Appropriate and timely resuscitation interventions can minimize brain damage. However, in cases of prolonged hypoxia (decreased oxygenation) there may be such long-term neurological problems involving seizures, mental retardation, cerebral palsy, or developmental delay.

Bronchopulmonary Dysplasia

Bronchopulmonary dysplasia (BPD) is a progressive chronic lung disease that is associated with prolonged use of oxygen and respiratory therapy used for RDS or other respiratory problems (Merritt, Northway, & Boyton, 1988; Ruiz, LaFever, Hakanson, Clark, & Williams, 1981). Infants who need mechanical oxygen therapy for more than 30 days are at-risk for developing BPD. Infants weighing less than 1250 grams at birth often develop BPD. The onset of BPD is characterized by increased oxygen requirements; emphysema results, and oxygenation is more difficult. Right lung failure may occur if the disease progresses. Infants with severe BPD often have respiratory problems for the first few years of life. It is not uncommon for these babies to be difficult feeders and to have overall developmental problems.

In premature infants BPD or chronic lung disease has been documented to be related to intellectual delay. Intellectual impairment shown to be associated with BPD is due to brain atrophy (Tay-Uyboco, Kwaitkowski, Cates, Kavanaugh, & Rigatto, 1989). This is the result of chronic hypoxia. In fact, the greater the infant's need for additional oxygen the greater the likelihood of neurodevelopmental delay (Nelson, 1991).

Perinatal Brain Damage

High-risk premature infants are vulnerable to brain damage that may contribute to later neurodevelopmental disorders. Several perinatal complications that result in disabilities are described below.

Intraventricular Hemorrhage

Intraventricular hemorrhage (IVH) is common in premature newborns. Generally IVH is more common among infants of low gestational age. Fifty percent of the premature infants with birthweights less than 1500 grams experience IVH. Symptoms of intraventricular hemorrhage include decreased respiration, decreased alertness, and lower heart rate. Infants may lose consciousness and enter a coma due to brain insult.

There are four grades of IVH injury (Grades I–IV). Grade IV is the most severe and involves severe bleeding into the ventricles and brain tissue (Papile, Burstein, Burstein, & Koffler, 1978). This results in lesions and asphyxia with decreased blood flow, which in turn compromise the infant's neurodevelopmental integrity. One of the major long-term sequela is cerebral palsy. The prognosis is dependent on the extent of intracranial pressure caused by the bleeding and the extent of the lesion damage, as well as the severity of complications such as bradycardia or cardiac arrest.

Follow-up studies have shown that Grades III and IV bilateral hemorrhages, that is hemorrhages on both sides of the brain, result in more major disabilities than unilateral hemorrhages (one side of the brain) (Nelson, 1991). This is because contralateral (opposite side) brain areas are able to assume control of the damaged areas. Most severe hemorrhages may injure the caudate nucleus, which is part of the basal ganglia of the brain. This injury is expressed in delayed developmental milestones, particularly a delay in walking. Visual attention deficits and poor visual motor function are typical of infants with more severe hemorrhage (Vohr et al., 1989). Many preterm infants with lower grades (I and II) IVH hemorrhages do not suffer later medical or developmental problems. Minor extracranial hemorrhages termed **cephalhematomas** are common in both term and preterm infants and do not usually result in deleterious results.

Intraventricular hemorrhage is now diagnosed with cranial ultrasounds. These imaging techniques are done weekly and in some units even daily to detect and follow cranial injuries. However, the predictive ability of the ultrasound techniques are limited because ultrasonography localizes the hemorrhage but it does not adequately evaluate the tissue damage. In addition other factors such as the infant's social environment and perinatal complications can influence the course of subsequent neurological development (Sostek, 1992)

■ STATE ORGANIZATION OF PRETERM INFANTS

Newborn Infant States

State behaviors begin during the fetal period. Between 26 and 28 weeks gestational age, cyclical periods of activity and quiet can be identified. As the fetus develops, these rest and activities periods involve more complex behaviors and by 32 weeks are distinguishable states (Fogel, 1991).

Newborn full-term infants typically show organized periods of sleep and alertness that appear with regularity. These periods are called infant **states** and are defined as relatively stable clusters of functional patterns and physiological variables that are organized and repeated over a 24-hour period (Prechtl & Beintema, 1968). Behavioral states reflect neonates' level of arousal, determine their reaction to the environment, and can be modified in response to external stimulation (Lenard, von Bernuth, & Prechtl, 1968). They are considered to be a reliable indicator of central nervous system integrity (Brazelton, 1973).

Through careful observation of newborns, Wolff (1966) identified six states that healthy full-term neonates typically exhibit in a 24-hour period. Developmental changes in the central nervous system modify sleeping, crying, and alert states.

The six states observed in full-term neonates include (Brazelton, 1973):

Quiet Sleep: The baby sleeps quietly with little or no movement. Breathing is regular, but the baby will startle to a loud noise.

Active Sleep: This phase is marked by REM sleep in which rapid eye movements are present. Eyelids flutter, gross body movements and facial grimaces are evident. Respiration is irregular.

Drowsy: This is a transitional state that occurs either before falling asleep or awakening. The eyelids slowly open and close, and there is increased body movement with irregular respirations.

Quiet Alert: In this state the baby is quiet with eyes open more than 15 seconds. Responsiveness to voices and faces is heightened. This is an optimum state for parent-infant interaction.

Active Alert: While the baby is alert and responsive to the environment, more body movement is evident. Often toward the end of this state there is some fussiness. Vocalizations are more typical of this phase.

Crying: This state may appear after any of the states but often occurs following the active alert period. Crying lasts for more than 15 seconds and is accompanied by arm and leg thrusts and skin color changes.

Infant state behavior is important for several reasons. States can be regulated by decreasing or increasing stimulation to infants. Parents who understand state regulation can transition their infant from one state to another to promote alertness, quieting, or assist self-regulating behaviors. This knowledge can enhance parents' feelings of self-esteem and competence. In addition, parents can develop a picture of their baby's individual rhythmicity by observing how long the baby spends in a particular state. This information is useful in reading a baby's caregiving cues and needs.

State behavior is also used in neonatal assessment. The widely used Brazelton Neonatal Behavioral Assessment Scale (NBAS), developed by T. Berry Brazelton (1973), measures infants' behavioral organization as well as their ability to transition across states. The NBAS considers the way that states change during the assessment and the variability of states as indicators of neurological functioning. The infants' ability for self-organization and calming are considered important for behavior (Rosenblith, 1992).

Preterm Infant State

Defining behavioral states in preterm infants is difficult because their neurologic integrity is still immature. This is particularly true of preterms whose gestational age is 35 weeks or less. Studies of preterms have shown generally that arousal, sleep, and crying states are more easily distinguished as the infants approach 40 weeks gestational age (Aylward, 1981). Let us turn first to the studies of states in normally developing fetuses and then to what is known about preterm infant states.

Among normally developing babies rhythmic periods of activity and sleep appear in the late fetal period (Johnson, Besinger, & Thomas, 1989; Robertson, 1987). Between 4 and 5 months, irregular periods of activity and rest begin to appear. Quiet sleep and REM sleep states can be detected in the 28-week fetus. Subsequently, there are regular patterns of quiet and activity that continue until birth (Sterman & Hoppenbrouwers, 1971). Between 34 and 38 weeks conceptual age the fetus shows organized levels of states that approximate states observed in newborns (Parmelee & Stern, 1972).

Depending on their level of maturity, preterm infants' states range from organized to minimally organized (Garbanti & Parmelee, 1987). In very early premature infants, 23 to 27 weeks, states are diffuse. At this age infants show jerky movements and irregular respiration and heart rate. During sleep, there are tremors and twitching movements as well as eye movements. Crying is infrequent and is not sustained long when it occurs.

Preterm infants between 30 and 37 weeks gestation gradually develop a quiet sleep state with an accompanying decrease in body movement and more regular respiration. Around 30 to 33 weeks, states are not clearly defined and typically show more in the way of transition-state activities (High & Gorski 1985). Transitional states are more difficult to identify in terms of observable behaviors. Behaviors that do appear occur only briefly or are fragmented.

Later, toward 37 weeks, states are more easily discerned. After 37 weeks heart rate, respiration, body movement, and eye movement become more closely aligned to the preterm's state. Nonintrusive observation of premature infants' state patterns are done by monitoring their physiological and behavioral changes. Infant monitoring equipment is linked to computers, which record the changes. In a computer-linked continuous observation study of preterm infants, High and Gorski (1985) found that with increasing gestational age, the total amount of sleep time decreased with a marked increase in the amount of time premature infants spent in awake states.

Garbanti and Parmelee (1987) conducted 24-hour microanalytic studies of individual state parameters of preterm infants in the NICU. This analysis looked at very subtle behavioral changes, not readily observed. They found distinct differences between younger, fragile infants compared to the older, healthier preterm infants. Younger sicker infants displayed more disorganized behaviors, heart rate, respiration, and body movements. Older infants showed more pronounced behaviors and consistently were more attuned to environmental stimuli as they matured.

High and Gorski (1985) expanded the newborn 6-state system to a 10-state system to better describe preterm infants' sleep/awake states. Their system includes transition state behaviors for preterm infants, which are seen more often than organized states. These behaviors, though brief, are usually precursors to more organized, clearly definable state behaviors. The addition of transition states means that appropriate developmental interventions can be planned better. Table 2–2 outlines the 10-state classification system.

Recognizing the elements of state behaviors is particularly useful when planning developmental care interventions for preterm infants.

TABLE 2–2. Preterm States and State Transitions

State		Descriptions
State 1	Quiet sleep	Eyes closed. No movement except startles. Regular respiration. Deep sleep state.
	Transition	Some rapid eye movement and motor movement
State 2	Active sleep	Rapid eye movements. Bursts of motor activity. Irregular respiration.
	Transition	Eyelids open and close briefly. Startles.
State 3	Drowsy	Transitional state. Eyes open and close. Irregular respirations. Increasing activity level.
	Transition	Increasingly fussy. More of the above, plus unsustained crying, grimacing, increase or decrease in color.
State 4	Quiet alert	Eyes half open for more than 15 seconds. Regular respirations. No body movements.
	Transition	Spurts of body movements. Color change.
State 5	Active awake	Eyes open. Much spontaneous activity. Irregular respirations. Irritable and active. Crying episodes are less than 15 seconds.
	Transition	Brief fussiness. Increased motor activity.
State 6	Crying	Sustained cry for more than 15 seconds. Color change to red. Average to high motor movements.
	Transition	To awake state. Motor movement decreases. Crying episodes decrease to less than 15 seconds.

Infants' level of arousal and physiologic and behavioral signs provide caregivers with information that can help them plan appropriate interventions. For example, the movements and responses of very fragile infants may well signal state disorganization and tell the caregiver that any unnecessary stimulation is unwarranted. Older, more intact preterm infants may have alert periods that provide opportunities for parent-infant interactive exchanges. Caregivers can, to some extent, manipulate the infants' state, particularly in older, stable prenatal infants. Repositioning infants or presenting auditory or visual stimuli can make an infant more alert and prepared for interactions with caregivers.

Read the following descriptions and identify the infant state.

Jennifer, a full-term newborn is awake and is quietly looking at objects in her environment. Her eyes are bright and shiny. What is this infant state? Explain?

Mr. and Mrs. Allen sit by the incubator in the NICU and watch their 38-week baby boy. His eyelids flutter, and he begins to move his arms. What state are they probably observing?

Kyle, a 26-week premature infant, lies in his isolette. His eyes are shut, and his body moves with jerks and tremors. What could you say about Kyle's state behaviors?

Joshua, a 37-week premature infant, is lying quietly in his crib. His eyes are shining, and he is focusing on a small toy placed near him. What behavioral signs would indicate Joshua is moving to another state?

Lynette, a 26-week premature infant, shows only a few tremors and movements sleeping. What would you say about this baby's state? What other state is Lynette likely to display?

■ BEHAVIORAL RESPONSITIVITY OF PRETERM INFANTS

When I first saw my baby, I was unprepared for the sight. She was so tiny! I could hardly see her for the tubes and machinery. She lay there with her eyes closed, her body twitching. With all that was going on around her she gave no response. It was hard for me to accept that she was my baby.

While the fetus is growing in the womb its physiologic functions are supported by the mother. The circulatory system, digestive processes, and temperature regulation are all maintained through the mother's body. The fetus floats in amniotic fluid within a dark, quiet womb. Premature birth brings sudden changes and physiologic demands on the infant. Because of their neurologic and physiologic immaturity, these infants are often unable to meet the demands placed upon them, consequently they become unstable (Bozynski et al., 1990). Medical interventions that entail drug therapy, surgery, or supporting machinery are required for stabilization.

Infants born earlier than 40 weeks show behavioral responses that differ from the responses of full-term infants. Strong reflexes that are normal among full-term infants are either weak or not present in preterm infants (Prechtl & Beintema, 1968). At 28 weeks the rooting, sucking, and swallowing reflexes can be elicited, but are slow. The coordination of these reflexes occurs at approximately 34 weeks (Fanaroff & Klaus, 1986). Reflex development reflects the neurological functioning of preterm infants. Als and others propose that integration and differentiation of neurological function evident in the developing preterm infant is guided through interactions with the environment (Als, 1983; Ayres, 1986).

Physiologic stability, responsiveness to external stimuli, and state behaviors generally vary greatly depending on the age and medical status of the baby. Compared to full-term infants, preterm infants are usually disorganized. Preterm infants are less responsive, less alert, and less active (Coll, Emmons, & Anderson, 1987). Their development, which is uneven through the neonatal period and the first few months of life, is accompanied by signs of distress such as heart rate deceleration, cyanosis, vomiting, or gagging (Goldberg & DiVitto, 1983).

A number of studies have documented that normally unresponsive fragile premature infants have intense, dramatic physiologic changes termed "overshoots" and become hyperresponsive in response to intense stimuli (Gorski, Krafchuk, Tronick, & Clifton, 1983). These physiological changes include decreased heart rate, decreased oxygen consumption, and increased irritability. Caregivers must assess the effects of stimuli levels on the preterm infant in order to maintain stable physiologic functioning.

■ SUMMARY

Advances in medical techniques for supporting life in fragile premature infants has resulted in decreased mortality and morbidity. As more vulnerable infants survive there is concern for their short- and long-term developmental outcomes. Premature infants with immature nervous systems must adapt to the extrauterine environment. Depending on their premature perinatal and postnatal experience they may develop chronic disabilities and behavior problems.

Normal labor occurs in three stages: Stage one is the longest phase and results in dilation and effacement of the cervix; stage two is marked by the birth of the fetus; stage three, the briefest stage, is characterized by expulsion of the placenta. The etiology of premature labor is still a mystery. What is known is that fragile premature infants may experience complications during labor and delivery.

Premature and low birthweight infants face problems that place them at-risk for development. The most frequent disorders include respiratory distress syndrome (RDS), apnea, asphyxia, and bronchopulmonary dysplasia.

Newborn full-term infants show organized patterns of behavior known as states. Six states that normally occur with regularity throughout a 24-hour period are quiet sleep, active sleep, drowsy, quiet alert, active alert, and crying. Preterm infants do not display clearly defined states. Rather, states are diffused and characterized by transitional state signs. As preterm infants develop and mature, their state behaviors become more distinct.

■ REFERENCES

Als, H. (1983). Infant individuality: Assessing patterns of very early development. In J. D. Call, E. Galenson, & R. L. Tyson (Eds.), *Frontiers in infant psychiatry* (pp. 363–378). New York: Basic Books.

Als, H. (1986). A synactive model of neonatal behavioral organization: Framework for assessment of neurobehavioral development in the premature infant and for the support of infants and parents in the neonatal intensive care environment. *Physical and Occupational Therapy in Pediatrics*, 6, 3–53.

Apgar, V. A. (1953). A proposal for a new method of evaluation of the new born infant. *Anesthesia and Analgesia*, 32, 260–267.

Aylward, G. P. (1981). The developmental course of behavioral states in preterm infants: A descriptive study. *Child Development*, 52, 564–568.

Ayres, J. (1986). *Southern California Sensory Integration Tests* (Rev.). Los Angeles: Western Psychological Services.

Babson, S. G., Benson, R. C., Pernoll, M. L. & Benda, G. I. (1980). Assessment of fetal health in high risk labor. In S. G. Babson & R. C. Benson (Eds.), *Management of high risk pregnancy in intensive care of the neonate* (pp. 22–41). St. Louis: C. V. Moseby.

Batshaw, M. L., & Perret, Y. M. (1986). *Children with handicaps: A medical primer*. Baltimore: Brookes.

Bozynski, M. E. A., DiPietro, M. A., Meisels, S. J., Plunkett, J. W., Burpee, B., & Claflin, P. (1990). Cranial sonography and neurological examination of extremely preterm infants. *Developmental Medicine and Child Neurology, 32*, 575–581.

Brazelton, T. B. (1973). *Neonatal behavioral assessment scale: Clinics in developmental medicine*. Philadelphia: Lippincott.

Challis, J. R. G., & Mitchell, B. F. (1981). Hormonal control of preterm and term parturition. *Seminars in Perinatology, 5*, 192–202.

Coll, C. G., Emmons, L., & Anderson, L. (1987). Behavioral responsivity in preterm infants. In N. Gunzenhauser (Ed.), *Infant stimulation* (pp. 64–71). Skillman, NJ: Johnson & Johnson.

Creasy, R. K., & Resnik, R. (1989). *Maternal-fetal medicine: Principles and practice* (2nd ed.). Philadelphia: W. B. Saunders.

Daze', A. M. (1985). Respiratory development and disease in the newborn. In A. M. Daze' & J. W. Scanlon (Eds.), *Neonatal nursing* (pp. 112–161). Baltimore: University Park Press.

Fanaroff, A., & Klaus, M. (1986). Feeding and selected disorder of the gastrointestinal tract. In M. Klause & A. Fanaroff (Eds.), *Care of the high-risk neonate* (pp. 113–146). Philadelphia: W. B. Saunders.

Fogel, A. (1991). *Infancy* (2nd ed.). New York: West Publishing Co.

Garbanti, J. A., & Parmelee, H. A. (1987). State organization in preterm infants: Microanalysis of 24-hour polygraph recording. In N. Gunzenhauser (Ed.), *Infant Stimulation* (pp. 51–64). Skillman, NJ: Johnson & Johnson.

Goldberg, S., & DiVitto, B. (1983). *Born too soon*. San Francisco: W. H. Freeman.

Gorski, P., Krafchuk, E. E., Tronick, E. Z., & Clifton, R. K. (1983). Behavioral and cardiac responses to the sound in preterm neonates varying in risk status: A hypothesis of their paradoxical reactivity. In T. M. Field & A. Sostek (Eds.), *Infants born at risk: Physiological, perceptual and cognitive process*. New York: Grune & Stratton.

High, D. C., & Gorski, P. (1985). Recording environmental influences on infant development in the intensive care nursery. In A. W. Gottfried & J. L. Gaiter (Eds.), *Infant stress under intensive care* (pp. 131–156). Baltimore: University Publishing.

Johnson, T. R. B., Besinger, R. E., & Thomas, R. L. (1989). The latest clues to fetal behavior and well-being. *Contemporary Pediatrics*, pp. 66–84.

Karim, S. M. M. (1968). Appearance of prostaglandin F2 in human blood during labor. *British Medical Journal, 4*, 618–621.

Kitchen, W., & Murton, L. J. (1985). Survival rates of infants with birth weight between 501 and 1,000g. *American Journal of Diseases of Children, 139*, 470–471.

Klaus, M. H., & Fanaroff, A. A. (1993). *Care of the high-risk Neonate* (4th, ed.). Philadelphia: W. B. Saunders.

Korones, S. B. (1986). *High-risk newborn infants*. St. Louis: C. V. Mosby.

Kumar, D., Goodno, J. A., & Barns, A. C. (1962). Isolation of progesterone from human pregnant myometrium. *Nature, 195*, 1204.

Lenard, H. G., Von Bernuth, H., & Prechtl, H. F. R. (1968). Reflexes and their relationship to behavioral state in the newborn. *Acta Paediatrica Scandinavica, 57*, 177–185.

Merritt, T. A., & Hallman, M. (1988). Surfactant replacement. A new era with many challenges for neonatal medicine. *American Journal of Diseases of Children, 142*, 1333–1339.

Merritt, T. A., Northway, W. H. Jr., & Boynton, B. R. (Eds.), (1988). *Bronchopulmonary dysplasia*. Boston: Blackwell Scientific.

Narayan, A. (1986). Complications in premature infants. *Postgraduate Medicine, 79*, 91–93, 96–101.

Nelson, M. N. (1991, November). *Vulnerabilities of high-risk infants: Origins and characteristics of perinatal brain damage*. Paper presented at Developmental Interventions in Neonatal Care Conference, Anaheim, California.

Papile, L,, Burstein, J., Burstein, R., & Koffler, H. (1978). Incidence and evolution of subependymal and intraventricular hemorrhage: A study of infants with birthweights less than 1500 grams. *Journal of Pediatrics, 92,* 529–534.

Parmelee, A. H. Jr., & Stern, E. (1972). Development of states in infants. In C. D. Clemete, D. P. Purpura, & F. E. Mayer (Eds.), *Sleep and the maturing nervous system.* New York: Academic Press.

Perelman, R. H., & Farrell, P. M. (1982). Analysis of causes of neonatal death in the United States with specific emphasis on fatal hyaline membrane disease. *Pediatrics, 70,* 570–575.

Philip, A. G. S. (1987). *Neonatalogy: A practical guide* (3rd ed.). Philadelphia: W. B. Saunders.

Prechtl, H. F. R., & Beintema, D. J. (1968). The neurological examination of the full-term infant. *Clinics in Developmental Medicine,* No. 28. London: International Medical Publication with Heinemann Medical.

Robertson, S. S. (1987). Human cyclic motility: Fetal-newborn continuities and newborn state differences. *Developmental Psychology, 20,* 425–445.

Rosenblith, J. (1992). *In the beginning* (2nd ed.). Newbury Park, CA: Sage.

Ruiz, M. P. D., LaFever, J. A., Hakanson, D. O., Clark, D. A., & Williams, M. L. (1981) Early development of infants at birthweight less than 1000 grams with reference to mechanical ventilation in newborn period. *Pediatrics, 68,* 330–335.

Shapiro, D. L. (1992). Surfactant replacement therapy. In R. A. Polin & W. W. Fox (Eds.), *Fetal and neonatal physiology* (6th ed., pp. 1007–1014). Philadelphia: W. B. Saunders.

Sostek, A. M. (1992). Prematurity as well as extraventricular hemorrhage influence on developmental outcome at 5 years. In S. L. Friedman & M. D. Sigman (Eds.), *The psychological development of low birthweight children* (pp. 259–274). Norwood, NJ: Ablex.

Sterman, M. B., & Hoppenbrouwers, T. (1971). The development of sleepwalking and rest activity patterns from fetus to adult in man. In M. B. Sterman, D. J. McGinty, & A. M. Adinolfi (Eds.), *Brain development and behavior* (pp. 203–228). New York: Academic Press.

Tay-Uyboco, J. S., Kwiatkowski, K., Cates, D. B., Kavanagh, L., & Rigatto, H. (1989). Hypoxic airway construction in infants of very low birthweight recovering from moderate to severe bronchopulmonary dysplasia. *Journal of Pediatrics, 115*(3), 456–459.

Vohr, B. R., Garcia-Coll, C., Mayfield, S., Brann, B., Shaul, P., & Oh, W. (1989) Neurologic and developmental status related to the evolution of visual-motor abnormalities from birth to two years of age in preterm infants with intraventricular hemorrhage. *Journal of Pediatrics, 115,* 296–302.

Wallenburg, H. C. S. (1983). Human labor. In R. Boyd & F. C. Battaglia (Ed.), *Perinatal medicine.* London: Butterworths International Medical Reviews.

Wolff, P. H. (1966). The causes, controls, and organization of behavior in the neonate. *Psychological Issues, 5,* 1–58.

■ CHAPTER 3

Preterm Infant Risk Conditions

*The role of the nurse is to put the patient in
the best state so that nature can act on him.*
Florence Nightingale

■ INTRODUCTION

Technological advances have dramatically improved the life chances of preterm infants. As a result there is a significant increase in the number of high-risk infants who survive the neonatal period. Infants born as early as 23 weeks gestation and weighing less than 500 grams now survive hospitalization (Buehler, Kleinman, Hogue, Strauss, & Smith, 1987). Bennett (1987) reported that between 1960 and 1980 the number of low birthweight infants doubled. But many of these infants are at risk for biological and psychosocial disabilities.

During the past 25 years, longitudinal studies of developmental outcomes for low birthweight and premature infants have shown that developmental problems are common in this population (Cohen & Beckwith, 1979; Hack & Farnoff, 1986). Between 10 to 20% of very low birthweight (VLBW) infants have major neurodevelopmental abnormalities associated with cerebral palsy, visual or hearing impairments, and mental retardation. Approximately 50% of VBLW infants manifest minor neurosensory problems such as delayed language, cognitive dysfunctions, attention disorders, emotional immaturity, and learning disabilities during preschool or early school years (Bennett, 1990).

The extent to which preterm infants develop optimally is determined by a complex interplay of environmental and biologic factors. Many factors place a premature infant at risk for development. Included are the degree of prematurity, quality of prenatal care, maternal health, and medical vulnerability. Other contributors to risk include psychosocial disadvantages such as teenage parents, poverty, poor parenting skills, and maternal substance abuse. Increasingly, data indicate that the NICU environment may adversely affect the physiological and behavioral stability of preterm infants. Even the routine care of premature infants in neonatal intensive care units may be stressful and present sensory overload for the infants. Very low birthweight (VLBW) or acutely ill infants may be particularly vulnerable to the physical and social features of the NICU environment.

Because of their neurologic immaturity and physiological instability, premature infants have a limited ability to adapt to the demands of a stressful external environment. Consequently, they can become overstimulated and show signs of medical distress. Infants show signs of stress to intrusive stimuli as well as make attempts to calm and regulate themselves. By assisting infants to self-regulate, caregivers ameliorate the risks neonates encounter in the NICU.

In this chapter we will first examine experiences that stress preterm infants. We will look at elements of the NICU environment and caregiving procedures that affect infants in the NICU. Next, the infants' signs of adapting to the environmental procedures will be outlined. Preventive interventions that can reduce the potentially harmful effects of the NICU environment and routine caregiving procedures will also be discussed.

■ THE NICU ENVIRONMENT

Risks

The neonatal intensive environment designed to medically sustain the fragile preterm infant is a sharp contrast to the peaceful intrauterine environment. The NICU environment may interfere with the premature infant's ability to develop, organize behavioral states, self-regulate, or integrate needed coping adaptations (Lawhon, 1986). Sick or fragile premature infants may experience bradycardia, decreased oxygenation, or sleep deprivation in response to stressful environmental stimulation.

Infants begin life in a quiet, modulated environment, the womb. While in the womb, they experience diurnal rhythms, regulated temperature, protection from loud sounds and light, and continuous tactile feedback from contact with the walls of the amniotic sac. Infants born prematurely are dramatically thrust from this peaceful environment into a noisy, brightly lit, intensive care environment. They must try to adapt to this intrusive environment. Their immaturity and physiologic instability make them particularly vulnerable to the onslaught of environmental stimulation as well as the ongoing medical interventions.

Since premature infants' sensory and motor systems are not well developed, they are often too fragile to tolerate stimulation. Their response to environmental stressors involves both behavioral and physiologic changes. These changes include color change, increased or decreased respiration rates, changes in oxygenation, arching, hypotonicity, irregular cardiac rates, and interruptions/changes in sleep-wake patterns (Lott, 1989). Because the extrauterine environment of the preterm infant is so different than that of the intrauterine environment, researchers have directed attention toward analyzing the effects of the NICU environment on premature infants (Blackburn & Patterson, 1991; Korner, 1987).

It used to be assumed that preterm infants were understimulated in the NICU (Korner, 1987). This was known as the Sensory Deprivation Model. In the 1960s researchers were concerned that preterm infants in isolettes experienced only white background noise and consequently lacked adequate stimulation for normal development (Rothchild, 1966). By the 1970s and 1980s researchers revised their view of a sensory deprivation model of the nursery environment and replaced it with an overstimulation model in the NICU environment. Investigators reported that the pattern of stimulation was inappropriate rather than an inadequate amount of stimulation in the NICU (Gorski, 1985; Lawson, Daum, & Turkewitz, 1977).

Subsequent analyses of caregiving in the NICU showed that far from being understimulated, preterm infants routinely experience overstimulation in intensive care (High & Gorski, 1985). In fact, the NICU experience is now considered potentially stressful to the infant (VandenBerg, 1985). Gorski (1984) has argued that many of the health problems faced by neonates in the NICU result from the newborn's attempt to adapt to the NICU environment and necessary medical procedures. Fragile preterm infants must cope with an environment characterized by bright lights, loud noise, frequent medical interventions, handling, and impersonal interactions while at the same time they are easily taxed by the intensive care environment.

Wolke (1987) reported that infants in the NICU are exposed to frequent handling and procedures in a day. VLBW infants experience 234 aversive procedures daily. Cardiac and respiration rates have been shown to increase in very ill infants in response to environmental stimulation (Catlett & Holditch-Davis, 1990). Environmental stress may trigger apnea episodes in acutely ill premature infants. Noise, light, and handling disrupts infant sleep states and causes premature infants to use energy needed for growth and development to cope with the deleterious stimuli (Peabody & Lewis, 1985). Other side effects such as recurrent apnea, postnatal intraventricular hemorrhage, and lung problems may result from neonatal intensive care (Lucey, 1984).

A major cause of state changes in hospitalized premature infants is medical and caregiving interventions. Frequent interventions, which may occur on average five times each hour, disrupt the infant's sleep (Catlett & Holditch-Davis, 1990). Studies of sleep deprivation in animals has shown such dramatic effects as permanently altered brain functioning, irritability, and altered sexual functioning in adulhood (Mirmiran, 1986). Denenberg and Thoman (1981) have shown that actual (REM) sleep is necessary for infant brain development. For acutely ill infants in the NICU, the reduction in quiet sleep may be harmful to their development.

When considering the impact of the NICU environment on the development of preterm infants, it is important to remember that this environment serves not only as a medical support for the infant but also as a backdrop for early social, emotional, and cognitive interactions. Unlike the home environment, which is often designed to foster developmental growth for the full-term infant, the NICU environmental demands may tax stable preterm infants' ability to respond even minimally to caregivers (Field, 1987). Further there is little in the way of contingent social interactions typically experienced by term infants (Gaiter, 1985). Heriza and Sweeney (1990) suggest that infants in the NICU receive the wrong kind of stimulation administered by the wrong person.

Parents, too, often perceive the NICU environment as stressful and overwhelming, which contributes to difficulties in establishing positive parent-infant interactions (Miles & Carter, 1983). It is generally agreed that parent-infant attachment and involvement of parents with their infants is adversely affected by many aspects of the NICU environment (Graven et al., 1992). Clinicians are concerned that parents who face multiple sources of stress, including guilt about the early birth, separation from their infant, and the ongoing medical crises, must also attempt to adapt to the overwhelming NICU environment (Perehudoff, 1990).

Some features of the neonatal intensive care nursery environment are:

- Constant lighting
- No significant diurnal light or rhythmic sound patterns
- Continuous white noise and muffled speech sounds in the incubator
- Unexpected loud noises
- Little rhythmic variation of animate or inanimate sensory experience

- Little contingent social interaction with stable infants
- Constant medical activity, much of it directed toward the infant

In the next section we will examine research on several aspects of the NICU environment. The focus is the short- and long-term effects of the environment on the well-being of the infant, as well as ways to modify the environment to promote the infant's optimal development.

Noise Levels in the NICU

High noise levels in the intensive care nursery are a major source of stress for infants. Careful analysis of the NICU environment shows that sound levels range from 45 to 80 decibels, with peaks at 120 decibels, levels equivalent to that produced by small machinery (Gottfried et al., 1981). Excessive sound levels result from monitor alarms, movement of medical equipment, radios, conversations, beepers, and telephone noise. This high NICU noise level is continuous and even increases during physicians' bedside rounds, admissions, or medical emergencies in the unit (Gottfried, 1985). Infants are usually not protected from the sounds, even in isolettes. Studies in which sounds in incubators are recorded reveal no sound muffling, (Bess, Peek, & Chapman, 1979; High & Gorski, 1985). Speech sounds, although heard inside isolettes, are indistinct (Weibley, 1989). When incubator doors are opened or closed the noise levels increase dramatically (Blennow, Svenningsen, & Almquist, 1974).

The noisy NICU environment affects premature infants (Lotas, 1992). In one study, observations of preterm infants during 2-hour periods indicated that loud noise resulted in physiological indicators of stress such as decreased oxygenation (TcPO2) of more than 10 points, increased heart rate, and 27 changes in infants' sleep and wake cycles (Catlett & Holditch-Davis, 1990). Ambient noise in the NICU has been found to affect intracranial pressure and transcutaneous oxygen tension in premature infants (Long, Alistair, Philip, & Lucey, 1980).

Hearing loss in adults has been shown to result from brief exposures to high noise levels of 80 decibels. Sensorineural deafness in premature infants may be related to the high sound levels in the NICU, although the noise level that is detrimental to preterm infants is still not established. Bergman et al. (1985) report that hearing loss occurs in 2.0 to 9.7% of premature infants in NICUs. It has been suggested that the combination of high sound levels with therapeutic levels of amnioglyoside and bilirubin frequently administered to premature infants may negatively affect auditory development. Clinical evidence has not supported that claim (deVries, Lary, & Dubowitz, 1985). Nevertheless, there is concern that persistent exposure to a noisy environment disrupts sleep states and interferes with other physiologic function.

Because full-term infants' sleep is usually disrupted after 3 minutes of sound levels of 75 dB or over, fragile premature infants exposed to excessive sound levels routinely experience state and sleep interruptions (Strauch, Brandt, & Edwards-Beckett, 1993). This is particularly disturbing because sleep of premature infants in the NICU is frequently disrupted, over 130 times in a 24-hour period (Korones, 1976). Consequently, premature infants experience sleep deprivation as a result of so little time spent in deep sleep, approximately 20 minutes per day. For acutely ill infants the lack of deep sleep may mean that they use energy needed for essential metabolic growth and healing (Graven et al., 1992; Lawhon, 1988).

Negative effects of noise stress have also been reported to affect medical staff in the NICU. In one study, neonatal nurses and physicians listened to an audiotape of the NICU sounds for an hour and reported headaches and feeling overwhelmed by the noise (Catlett & Holditch-Davis, 1990). Recent investigation of the effects of instituting a quiet hour during the 7-hour work shift found that medical staff and parents in the NICU reported decreases in their own stress levels (Strauch et al., 1993).

Light Levels in the NICU

In most neonatal intensive care units intense, cool white fluorescent lights are on throughout the 24-hour day. Studies of the light intensity in NICUs have shown that the average light intensity level ranges from 60 to 75 footcandles (Glass et al., 1985). The American Academy of Pediatrics' 1992 *Guidelines For Perinatal Care* recommends that lighting in the NICU be 60 footcandles. Although there is no documented evidence of the effects of ambient fluorescent lights on premature infants, research on animals, older children, and adults indicate a number of deleterious effects including chromosomal breakage and alterations in biological rhythms and endocrine functions (Peabody & Lewis, 1985).

Glass and colleagues asked the question whether the standard bright lighting of the NICU might contribute to retinopathy of prematures (ROP). Low birthweight infants in a nursery with regular lighting (60 footcandles) were compared to infants of small birthweight in a nursery with reduced lighting (25 footcandles) during the duration of their hospital stay. They found significantly more retinopathy in the sample exposed to bright lights with a 30% greater incidence for infants weighing less than 1000 grams at birth. A further investigation of nursery illumination and ROP found that ROP onset occurs in the areas of the retina receiving the highest exposure to light (Fielder, Robinson, Shau, Ng, & Moseley, 1992). These preliminary findings point to exposure to continuous bright lights as a possible risk factor, but further studies are required to determine if early exposure to bright light levels is a causative factor in the development of ROP.

One study found that premature infants weighing less than 1000 grams who are exposed to the light intensity levels in the NICU have an increased incidence of retinopathy (Messner, 1972). Gibson et al. (1990) linked the increase of retinopathy with the increased survival of smaller infants. These findings have led several researchers to suggest that continuous light in the intensive care nursery is detrimental and induces sleep deprivation and changes in diurnal rhythms in infants (Peabody & Lewis, 1985).

Shogan and Schumann (1993) examined the relationship of oxygen saturation of sleeping infants between 26 and 37 weeks gestation to changes in environmental illumination in the NICU. Rapidly increasing illumination was found to elicit stressful responses in the infants. Lawson and Turkewitz (1986) found that premature infants in brightly lit NICUs kept their eyes closed more than other infants. For more stable preterm infants, this shut down may interfere with experiences and interactions needed for optimal development.

Preterm infants do not experience alternating day and night cycles typically experienced by full-term newborn infants in the home environment because lights are on 24 hours daily in most NICUs. Some investigators think that the absence of diurnal light cycles may interfere with normal biologic rhythms. Animal studies of the effects of continuous lighting indicate negative physical and biochemical effects, as well as growth retardation (Gottfried & Gaiter, 1985). Similarly, concerns have been raised regarding the effects of lack of cycled light on state and sleep patterns of preterm infants (Anders & Keener, 1985; Blackburn & Patterson, 1991).

■ MODIFYING THE NICU ENVIRONMENT

Healthy full-term infants are typically hospitalized for 1 to 4 days after birth. Their experience is in sharp contrast to fragile premature infants who are hospitalized an average of 28 days (Holmes et al., 1982). Their prolonged hospitalization is in an environment that is qualitatively different than the home environment. Outcomes for high-risk infants are believed to result from a multiplicity of factors that interact on the developing infant; such factors include the severity of neonatal morbidity, degree of physiological immaturity, medical complications, and the environmental conditions experienced in the intensive care unit. In this section we will examine ways to modify the NICU to promote optimal premature infant development.

Gorski, (1987) points out that the NICU is designed to manage the survival needs of preterm infants including respiration, nutrition, and thermal regulation but their long-term developmental needs are not addressed. These developmental needs include providing appropriate sensory feedback to the maturing central nervous system, fostering reciprocal and synchronous parent-infant interactions (see Figure 3–1), and providing appropriate response to infant states and biorhythms. Although medical intervention strategies have dramatically increased the survival rate of medically fragile infants, there are increased concerns about the prevalence of short-term and long-term neurodevelopmental disabilities.

The intensive care nursery can be intrusive and excessively stimulating; it also may provide disjunctive stimulation that is not contingent on the infant's behavior, making it difficult for preterm infants to cope with the various environmental demands of the NICU. Very low birthweight infants, because of their physiological and neurological immaturity, are particularly sensitive to the NICU environment. Investigators agree that the neonatal intensive care environment must be modified in order to reduce potential harm to the high-risk infant (Anderson, 1986; Bennett, 1990; Lester & Tronick, 1990).

In the past two decades, research and clinical practice have been directed at finding strategies that reduce preterm infant stress while at the same time creating a supportive environment for infants and their families (O'Donnell, 1990). Interventions have focused on noise reduction, light control, appropriate handling procedures, and family support. The effectiveness and outcomes of these interventions must still be systematically examined in order to determine "best practice."

Decreasing NICU Noise

Infants in NICUs receive large amounts of ongoing auditory stimulation for prolonged time periods (Thomas, 1989). The overall noise level in NICUs can be significantly reduced through individual actions of those entering the unit or through more systemic or global change. Individual staff members can decrease noise in several ways. They can monitor their conversations with other adults and encourage quiet talk by families and other staff members. NICU staff can respond to monitors quickly and drape incubators to muffle sounds.

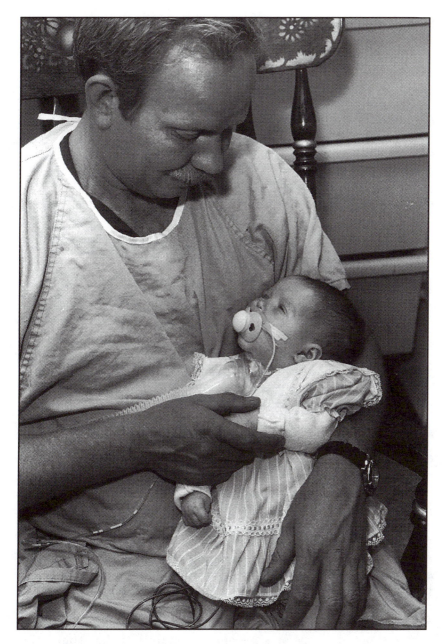

FIGURE 3-1. A father holding his daughter. (Photograph courtesy of Children's Hospital of Buffalo Department of Medical Photography.)

Routine delivery of medical and caregiving interventions can be designed to modify noise levels.

Inservice training can be used to inform staff of existing noise levels as well as the effects of a noxious audiological environment on fragile infants. Videotapes or audiotapes documenting routine unit activities can be used in inservice programs to present "first hand" the noise in the unit. Types of extraneous auditory stimulation should be considered in terms of their impact on infant, families, and staff. Units need to allow time for staff to plan ways to reduce unit sound levels.

Some unnecessary noise can be eliminated in the NICU by the following interventions:

- Lower Monitor alarms
- Limit conversations by infants' bedside
- Conduct physician and nurse rounds away from bedside
- Avoid dropping the mattress head
- Close isolette doors quietly
- Do not tap isolette
- Respond quickly to monitor alarms
- Muffle telephone bells, computer printers, and garbage lids
- Turn off radios in the unit
- Place fragile infants away from high traffic areas
- Post signs by infant's bed side such as "Quiet! I'm Sleeping"
- Purchase equipment, for example, incubators and alarms with low sound settings

VandenBerg, Gorski, and Brazelton (1988) have suggested a Quiet Hour protocol to minimize noise in intensive care units. Zahr (1994) used ear muffs over the ears of low birthweight premature infants to reduce noise intensity in the NICU. Compared to control infants, the infants with earmuffs had significantly higher mean oxygen saturation as well as less fluctuation in levels of oxygen saturation. These infants also spent more time in quiet sleep states. Catlett and Holditch-Davis (1990) suggest that the use of quiet, repetitive sounds to facilitate infant development should only be done with physiologically stable infants. Intermittent stimulation such as music boxes or tapes of parents' voices should be used only after carefully assessing the infant's ability to tolerate these sounds. If the infant shows signs of stress or physiologic instability, the stimulation should be discontinued.

Reducing Light Stress

Preterm infants are cared for in neonatal units that are continuously lit. Several researchers have expressed concern about the effect of lack of diurnal light cycles and artificial light on the sleep states of the neonates (Glass & Avery, 1987; Sheldon & Bell, 1987). Although there is documentation that sleep/wake cycles of premature infants are disrupted by 24-hour daylight, the long-term effects of light on the developmental outcomes of preterm infants are virtually unknown.

Because sleep problems are problematic in premature infant care, investigators have looked at the effects of day/night light cycles on the behaviors and sleep patterns of preterm infants. Blackburn and Patterson (1991) found that systematic day/night light levels resulted in significantly lower heart rates and overall activity levels in premature infants compared to infant groups in continuous light. Mann, Haddow, Stokes, Goodley, and Rutter (1986) reported that preterm infants who experienced reduced light and noise intensities between 7 PM and 7 AM, gained more weight, had significantly more sleep, and took less feeding time than their counterparts in continuous light. These findings suggest that NICU staff should work to establish day/night light levels in neonatal units to promote a developmentally supportive environment.

Although further research is needed on effects of light exposure on critical care neonates, lighting in most NICUs remains at high levels, especially during the day. Immature preterm infants may be stressed by the light levels, which in turn results in state disruption and behavioral disorganization (Als, 1986). Staff need to assess the optimum lighting necessary to support and enhance individual infants' biologic rhythms and still allow for good medical care.

NICU practitioners have suggested a number of interventions which include:

- Place blanket or cover over isolette or radiant warmers of more stable infants
- Use partial drape covering head/neck areas with acutely ill babies who need to be observed frequently by staff
- Move stable babies to unit areas where day/night light cycles are possible
- Institute light dimming periods in the unit
- Use individualized lighting at bedsides if feasible.

Although visual protection is needed for acutely ill infants, NICU health providers must assess the individual infant's tolerance and developmental changes when planning visual protection or stimulation. As infants mature they are able to tolerate more visual input. Older, more stable infants may be able to visually explore toys or mobiles placed within view. Face-to-face interactions during feeding or alert time can be appropriate visual stimulation. It is essential that NICU caregivers respond to infants' cues of stress overload and at those times discontinue visual stimulation.

■ MEDICAL AND CAREGIVING EXPERIENCES IN THE NICU

The first priority of NICU staff is the well-being of the infant. Various medical and nursing procedures such as ventilation, examination, and intubation are designed to meet the basic care needs of the premature infant. Many of these procedures involve continuous monitoring of the infant to assess their effectiveness. There is growing evidence that even routine procedures may have the net effect of adversely affecting the neonate.

Neonatal researchers have begun to investigate the stressful effects of specific treatment procedures and caregiving activities. These studies document infant stress responses to the medical treatments necessary to infant survival (Field, 1987). Peters (1992) found frequent periods of hypoxia, hyperoxia, and increased intracranial pressure (ICP) to be associated with routine nursing procedures including taking vital signs, position change of infant, removing transcutaneous probes, weighing infant, diaper change, routine radiographic examinations, adhesive surface removal, and suctioning. In those procedures associated with pain and discomfort, premature infants have increased heart rate and decrease in oxygenation (Catlett & Holditch-Davis, 1990).

Handling

There is increased concern that preterm infants regularly experience excessive handling. As Peters (1992) stated "the amount of infant disturbances has increased while the average birthweight and gestational age of infants treated in NICUs have decreased dramatically" (p. 79).

Investigators have found that premature infants are frequently handled as part of care by NICU health providers. Sixty to 70% of the contacts with premature infants are by nurses (Duxbury, Henly, Broz, Armstrong, & Wachdorf, 1984). Korones (1976) was the first to report that premature infants can experience 132 contacts involving handling over a 24-hour period. In their observations of sick infants, Gottfreid and Hodgman (1984) found that infants received up to 100 contacts in 24 hours. Peters (1992) reported 120 to 245 contacts per 24 hours.

Duxbury et al. (1984) found that average frequency of contacts per hour was 2.13, with a mean duration of these contacts 8.5 minutes. Compared to nonventilated infants, ventilated infants were exposed to longer and more frequent contacts. In contrast, Gaiter, Avery, Temple, Johnson, and White (1981) found no significant difference in handling related to an infant's acuity.

A majority of infants who enter the NICU have respiratory distress and require supplemental oxygen. Without satisfactory levels of oxygen infants experience hypoxia, which is a sequela of brain injury. Maintenance of sufficient oxygenation requires frequent handling of the neonate. Excessive handling during routine care for infants with respiratory distress syndrome is associated with periods of hypoxia. A number of studies have shown that preterm infants respond immediately to touch, and the response is often hypoxia (Beaver, 1987; Evans, 1991; Long, Alistair, Phillip, & Lucey, 1980).

Routine medical procedures such as heelsticks, intubation, and handling during diapering or repositioning after a medical intervention have been found to result in increased heart rate and decreased oxygenation (TcPO2) (Long et al., 1980; Morrow et al., 1991). Frequent handling in the NICU has been associated with the potential for intraventricular hemorrhage (Bada et al., 1990). For very premature infants, any type of touch can evoke stress responses (Beaver, 1987).

Sleep/State Disruptions

Because of the many care procedures administered daily, sleep of the critically infant is disrupted. Duxbury et al. (1984) found that infants who were most critically ill were disturbed more frequently and for longer time periods than more intact infants. Sick infants in their study were awakened every 38 minutes. To counter the frequent disruptions associated with care procedures, the authors recommend clustering caregiving activities to minimize disruption and promote longer sleep duration.

Neonatal state is defined as a set of organized behaviors that occur spontaneously and recur cyclically. Full-term infants have clearly defined states which reflect central nervous system integrity. Newborn states are sleep-wake cycles that include active sleep, quiet sleep, drowsiness, active alert, quiet alert, and crying. Stall organization is determined by endogenous factors and environmental influ-ences. The critical period during which states emerge are 32 to 36 weeks post conceptual age (Parmelee, Wenner, Akiyama, Schultz, & Stern, 1967).

The intensive care environment has been shown to be disruptive to the development of behavior states in premature infants (Lawson, Daum, & Turkewitz, 1977). Fajardo, Browning, Fisher, and Paton (1990) studied spontaneous states and state-relevant behaviors of 32- to 36-week-old infants in two different nursery environments. They found that a nursery environment with diurnal cycles and state-con-tingent nursing procedures promoted steadiness and duration of sleep states in infants. Thus, an important intervention for promot-ing the emergence of organized states is providing a nondisruptive NICU environment.

■ SIGNS OF PREMATURE INFANT STRESS AND SELF-REGULATION

Premature infants attempt to cope with the stimulation of bright lights, alarms, loud sounds of machines, and human voices in the NICU. To protect themselves from the demands of the external envi-ronment, they exhibit defensive behaviors. Signs of stress and self-regulation are the infant's signals to their caregivers that they are attempting to avoid or cope with environmental stressors.

Signs of Stress

When newborns in the NICU are overloaded by environmental and caregiving events, they show many behavioral manifestations of stress. These are sometimes called "time-out" signals (Als, 1986).

These signs of stimulus overload may be behavioral signs or physiological changes. They indicate that the infant needs time out from further stimulation. Signs of stimulus overload include:

- Turning away or turning the head
- Grimacing or putting the lips together
- Frowning or smiling
- Twitching motor movements
- Movement of arms, legs, and trunk
- Oxygen desaturation
- Arching of trunk, arm, neck
- Extending arms to one side, asymmetrically
- Fingers or toes splayed

- Shutting eyes
- Spitting up
- Drooling
- Changing respiration rate
- Moving bowels
- Changing color
- Seizures
- Vomiting
- Change in heart rate
- Yawning
- Going limp
- Tongue thrusts
- Hand-on-face maneuver
- Sighing

All of these stress signs may not appear in every infant. Their appearance will depend on the individual infant and the type of stimulus present. Some infants might be stressed by an auditory stimulus, whereas another may be stressed by a visual stimulus. Sensory input is not random but individualized according to each infant's tolerance.

Signs of Self-Regulation

Although infants exhibit behaviors that are indicators of stress, they also show signs of self-regulation or organization (Duffy & Als, 1989). These behaviors are calming for infants and help them to recover from stressors. It is important for NICU health personnel and parents to know and use these signs to promote infants' abilities to attain stability.

Certain infant signs and behaviors indicate that preterm infants are trying to shut out intense stimulation and calm themselves. This happens when the infant's central nervous system is unable to regulate incoming stimulation. The infant becomes hyperaroused and shows increased efforts to organize motor and physiologic systems to reach a quiet state. This attempt to return to a homeostasis is known as self-regulation. Self-regulation efforts may tax the infant's energies, particularly if the infant has difficulty calming down. Some signs of neonates' attempts to regulate themselves are:

- Hand-to-mouth movements
- Sucking
- Flexion
- Sneezing
- Yawning

- Gaze aversion
- Hiccuping
- Move to containment
- Shutting eyes
- Covering eyes or ears
- Hand-feet clasp

By recognizing these behaviors, medical care providers can assist infants' self-regulation by reducing stimulation or implementing strategies to facilitate the self-regulation process. For example, bedrolls can be used to surround infants who need containment. Sucking can be encouraged with a pacifier. Appropriately positioning an infant can provide motor stability or shut out environmental input.

■ CAREGIVING INTERVENTIONS

NICU health providers are reexamining their care interventions with attention to their effects on premature infants (Velasco-Whetsell, Evans, & Wang, 1992). The timing, frequency, and level of intrusiveness of the care procedures are being studied to determine effective ways for identifying and reducing stressful stimuli in the neonate's environment. VandenBerg (1985) points out that caregivers must carefully observe each infants' behavioral cue to each environmental event. Signs of infant stress and self-regulation need to be identified so that stimulation or caregiving responses can be modified to appropriately match the infant's level of organization and behavioral capacities.

Minimal handling protocols have been adopted in many NICUs (Langer, 1990). These protocols are designed to guide NICU health providers to deliver supportive and high quality care to fragile prematures who are unable to tolerate stress and routine procedures. The protocol directs medical and nursing interventions to implement proper positioning, comfort measures such as swaddling, and to implement care procedures based on individual assessment of infants' tolerance for contact.

Evans (1991) has suggested that NICU caregivers implement procedures to minimize excessive handling of fragile infants. These include allowing infants rest periods to recover following medical and caregiving procedures, placing signs on isolettes to alert staff to minimal handling policies, and employing individualized care plans.

Caregiving activities such as feeding or diapering with the full-term infant are usually coupled with smiles, gentle touch, or talk directed at the infant. In contrast, preterm infants are frequently handled during medical interventions; yet these interventions are generally not accompanied by soothing or comforting techniques. Even when infants are more stable and able to tolerate social exchanges, there are few social interactions linked with medical or caregiving interventions. In addition, caregiving activities in the NICU, such as feeding, usually are not temporally patterned nor tied to the infant's state or behavior (Blackburn, 1983). Individualized assessments of infants' maturation level, tolerance of stimulation, and response to stimuli are now used to plan appropriate developmental interventions in the NICU (Lester & Tronick, 1990; VandenBerg, 1990).

■ SUMMARY

The dramatic reduction in premature infant mortality has raised concern over the concomitant increase in handicapping conditions. Between 5 to 10% of premature/low birthweight infants have major handicaps. There are also reports of increases in more subtle handicaps that encompass learning disabilities, behavior disorders, and neurosensory deficits.

Premature infants are neurologically immature, consequently they often have difficulty adapting to the intrusive NICU environment. This environment is characterized by bright lights, noise, and repeated medical and caregiving interventions. In their effort to cope with this extrauterine environment, preterm infants attempt to self-regulate themselves physiologically. Often, they display signs of stress. Sensitive caregivers must learn to read both the signs of self-regulation and stress in order to modify their caregiving regimen.

Clinicians are investigating ways to ameliorate the noise and light in the neonatal nursery. Further, studies show that caregiving and medical interventions can be altered to assist infants to successfully manage these procedures.

■ REFERENCES

Als, H. (1986). A synactive model of neonatal behavioral organization: Framework for the assessment of the neurobehavioral development of the premature infant and his parents in the environment of the neonatal intensive care unit. *Physical and Occupational Therapy in Pediatrics, 6,* 3–55.

Anders, T. F., & Keener, M. (1985). Developmental course of nighttime sleep-wake patterns in full term and premature infants during the first year of life, I. *Sleep, 8,* 173–192.

Anderson, J. (1986). Sensory intervention with the preterm infant in the neonatal intensive care unit. *American Journal of Occupational Therapy, 40,* 19–26.

Bada, H. S., Korones, S. B., Perry, E. H., Arheart, K. L., Pourcyrons, M., Runyan, J. W., Anderson, G. D., Magill, H. L., Fitch, C. W., & Somes, G. W. (1990). Frequent handling in the neonatal intensive care and intraventricular hemorrhage. *Journal of Pediatrics, 117*, 126–131.

Beaver, P. K. (1987). Premature infants' response to touch and pain: Can nurses make a difference? *Neonatal Network 6* 13–17.

Bennett, F. C. (1987). Infants at biological risk. In M. J. Guralnick & F. C. Bennett (Eds.), *Effectiveness of early intervention for at-risk and handicapped children* (pp. 79–112). New York: Academic Press.

Bennett, F. C. (1990). Recent advances in developmental intervention for biologically vulnerable infants. *Infants and Young Children, 3*, 33–40.

Bergman, I., Friar, T., Hirsch, R., Holzman, I., Painter, M., & Shapiro, S (1985). Cause of hearing loss in the high-risk premature infant. *Pediatrics, 106*, 95–101.

Bess, F. H., Peek, B. F., & Chapman, J. J. (1979). Further observations on noise levels in infant incubators. *Pediatrics, 63*(1), 100–106.

Blackburn, S. (1983). Fostering behavioral development of high-risk infants. *Journal of Obstetrics, Gynecology and Neonatal Nursing, 12*, 76–85.

Blackburn, S., & Patterson, D. (1991). Effects of cycled light on activity state and cardiorespiratory function in preterm infants. *Journal of Perinatal and Neonatal Nursing, 4*, 47–54.

Blennow, G., Svenningsen, N. W., & Almquist, B. (1974). Noise levels in infant incubators (adverse effects?). *Pediatrics 53*, 29–32.

Buehler, J. W., Kleinman, J. C., Hogue, C. J. R., Strauss, L. T., & Smith, J. C. (1987). Birthweight-specific infant mortality, United States, 1960 and 1980. *Public Health Reports, 102*, 151–161.

Catlett, A. T., & Holditch-Davis, D. (1990). Environmental stimulation of the acutely ill premature infant: Physiological effects and nursing implications. *Neonatal Network, 8*, 19–26.

Cohen, S. E., & Beckwith, L. (1979). Preterm infant interaction with the caregiver in the first year of life and competence at age 2. *Child Development, 50*, 767–776.

Denenberg, V. H., & Thoman, E. B. (1981). Evidence for a functional role for active (REM) sleep in infancy. *Sleep, 4*, 185–191.

deVries, L. S., Lary, S. D., & Dubowitz, L. M. S. (1985). Relationship of serum bilirubin levels to ototoxicity and deafness in high-risk low birthweight infants. *Pediatrics, 76*, 351–354.

Duffy, F., & Als, H. (1989). Brain organization in infants: Electrical activity mapping. In N. Paul (Ed.), *Research in infant assessment* (pp. 33–46). White Plains, NY: March of Dimes Birth Defects Foundation.

Evans, J. C. (1991). Incidence of hypoxemia associated with caregiving in premature infants. *Neonatal Network, 10*, 17–24.

Fajardo, B., Browning, M., Fisher, D., & Paton, J. (1990). Effect of nursery environment or state regulation on very-low-birthweight premature infants. *Infant Behavior and Development, 13*, 287–303.

Field, T. (1987). Alleviating stress in ICU neonates. In N. Guzenhauser (Ed.), *Infant Stimulation: For whom, what kind, when and how much?* (pp. 121–129). Skillman, NJ: Johnson & Johnson.

Fielder, A. R., Robinson, J. Shau, D. E., Ng, K. Y., & Moseley, M. J. (1992). Light and retinopathy of prematurity: Does retinal location offer a clue? *Pediatrics, 89*, 648–653.

Gaiter, J. (1985). The behaviors and caregiving experiences of full term and preterm infants. In A. W. Gottfried & J. L. Gaiter (Eds.), *Infant stress under intensive care* (pp. 55–82). Baltimore: University Park Press.

Gaiter, J., Avery, G. G., Temple, C., Johnson, A., & White, N. (1981). Stimulation characteristics of nursery environments for critically ill preterm infants and infant behavior. In L. Stern, B. Salle, & B. Friis-Hansen (Eds.), *Intensive Care in the Newborn III* (pp 389–410). New York: Masson Publishing Company.

Glass, P., & Avery, G. (1987). Reply to Sheldon & Bell. *Pediatrics, 79*, 1053.

Glass, P., Avery, G. B., Subramanian, K. N. S., Keys, M. P., Sostek, A. M., & Friendly, D. S. (1985). Effect of bright light in the hospital nursery on the incidence of retinopathy of prematurity. *The New England Journal of Medicine, 313*, 401–404.

Gorski, P. (1985). Behavioral and environmental care: New frontiers in neonatal nursing. *Neonatal Network, 3*, 8–11.

Gorski, P. (1987, October). *Latest advances in neonatal medicine; Resultant neurodevelopmental opportunities and risks.* Paper presented at Developmental interventions in Neonatal Care Conference, Danville, CA.

Gorski, P., Hole, W., Leonard, C., & Martin, J. (1983). Direct computer recording of premature infants and nursery care. *Pediatrics, 72*, 198–202.

Gorski, P. A. (1984). Premature infant behavioral and physiological responses to caregiving intervention in the intensive care nursery. In J. D. Call, E. Galenson, & R. L. Tyson (Eds.), *Frontiers in infant psychiatry* (pp 142–169). New York: Basic Books.

Gottfried, A. W. (1985). Environment of newborn infants in special care units. In A. W. Gottfried & J. L. Gaiter (Eds.), *Infant stress under intensive care: Environmental neurology* (pp. 23–54). Baltimore: University Park Press.

Gottfried, A. W., & Gaiter, J. L. (1985). *Infant stress under intensive care.* Baltimore: University Park Press.

Gottfried, A. W., Wallace-Land, P., Sherman-Brown, S., King, J., Coen, C., & Hodgman, J. E. (1981). Physical and social environment of newborn infants in special care units. *Science, 214*, 673–675.

Graven, S. N., Bowen, F. W., Brooten, D., Eaton, A., Graven, M. N., Hack, M., Hall, L. A., Hansen, N., Hurt, H., Kavalhuna, R., Little, G. A., Mahan, C., Morrow, G., III, Oehler, J. M., Poland, R., Ram, B., Sauve, R., Taylor, P. M., Ward, S. E., & Sommers, J. G. (1992). The high risk infant environment part 1. The role of the neonatal intensive care unit in the outcome of high risk infants. *Journal of Perinatology, 12*(2), 164–172.

Hack, M., & Farnoff, A. A. (1986). Changes in the delivery room care of the extremely small infant (<750g): Effects on morbidity and outcome. *New England Journal of Medicine, 314*, 660–664.

Heriza, C. B., & Sweeney, J. K. (1990). Effects of NICU intervention on preterm infants: Part 1: Implications for neonatal practice. *Infants and Young Children, 2*(3), 31–48.

High, D. C., & Gorski, P. (1985). Recording environmental influences on infant development in the intensive care nursery. In A. W. Gottfried & J. L. Gaiter (Eds.), *Infant stress under intensive care* (pp. 131–156). Baltimore: University Park Press.

Holmes, D. L., Nagy, J. N., Slaymaker, F., Sosnowski, R. J., Prinz, S. M., & Pasternak, J. F. (1982). Early influences of prematurity, illness and prolonged hospitalization on infant behavior. *Developmental Psychology, 18*, 744–750.

Korner, A. F. (1987). Infant stimulation: Issues of theory and research. In N. Gunzenhauser (Ed.), *Infant stimulation: For whom, what kind, when, and how much?* (pp. 88–97). Skillman, NJ: Johnson & Johnson.

Korones, S. (1976). Disturbance and infant's rest. In T. Moore (Ed.), *Iatrogenic problems in NICU : Report of the 69th Ross Conference of Pediatric Research* (pp. 74–97). Columbus, OH: Ross Laboratories.

Korones, S. B. (1976). Disturbance and infants' rest. In T. D. Moore (Ed.), *Iatrogenic problems in neonatal intensive care: Resport of the Sixty-Ninth Ross Conference on Pediatric Research* (pp. 94–97). Columbus, OH.: Ross Laboratories.

Langer, V. S. (1990). Minimal handling protocol for the intensive care nursery. *Neonatal Network, 9*, 23–27.

Lawhon, G. (1986). Management of stress in premature infants. In D. J. Angelini, C. M. Whelan-Knapp, & R. M. Gibes (Eds.), *Perinatal/Neonatal nursing: A clinical handbook* (pp. 319–328). Boston: Blackwell Scientific Publications.

Lawhon, G. (1988, November). *Developmental intervention: Nursery issues and applications*. Paper presented at the National Conference for Developmental Intervention in Neonatal Care, San Diego, CA.

Lawson, K., Daum, C., & Turkewitz, G. (1977). Environmental characteristics of a neonatal intensive care unit. *Child Development, 48*, 1633–1639.

Lawson, K. R., & Turkewitz, G. (1986). [Letter to the Editor]. *New England Journal of Medicine, 314*, 449.

Lester, B. M., & Tronick, E. (Eds.). (1990). Introduction: Guidelines for stimulation with preterm infants. *Clinics in Perinatology: Stimulation and the Preterm Infant, 17*, xiii–xvii.

Long, J. G., Alistair, G. S., Philip A. G. S., & Lucey, J. F. (1980). Excessive handling as a cause of hypoexmia. *Pediatrics 65*, 203–206.

Lotas, M. J., (1992). Effects of light and sound in the neonatal intensive care unit environment on the low birthweight infant. *NAACOG'S Clinical Issues in Perinat & Women's Health Nursing, 3*, 34–44.

Lott, J. W. (1989. Developmental care of the preterm infant. *Neonatal Network, 7*, 21–28.

Lucey, J. F. (1984). The sleeping, dreaming fetus meets the intensive care nursery. In C. C. Brown (Ed.), *The many facets of touch* (pp. 75–81). Skillman, NJ: Johnson & Johnson.

Mann, N. P., Haddow, R., Stokes, L., Goodley, S., & Rutter, N. (1986). Effect of night and day on preterm infants in a newborn nursery: Randomised trial. *British Medical Journal, 29*, 1265–1267.

Messner, K. H. (1972). Light toxicity to the newborn retina. *Pediatric Research 12*, 530.

Miles, M. S., & Carter, M. C. (1983). Assessing parent stress in intensive care units. *American Journal of Maternal Child Nursing, 8*, 354–359.

Mirmiran, M. (1986). The importance of fetal/neonatal REM sleep. *European Journal of Obstetrics, Gynecology and Reproductive Biology, 21*, 283–291.

Morrow, C. J., Field, T. M., Scafidi, F. A., Roberts, J., Eisen, L., Larson, S. K., Hogan, A. E., & Bandstra, E. S. (1991). Differential effects of message and heelstick procedures on transcutaneous oxygen in preterm neonates. *Infant Behavior and Development, 14*, 397–414.

O'Donnell, J. (1990). The development of a climate for caring: A historical review of premature care in the United States from 1979 to 1990. *Neonatal Network, 8*, 7–17.

Parmelee, A. H., Wenner, W. H., Akiyama, Y., Schultz, M., & Stern, E. (1967). Sleep states in premature infants. *Developmental Medicine and Child Neurology, 9*, 70–77.

Peabody, J. C., & Lewis, K. (1985). Consequences of newborn intensive care. In A. W. Gottfried & J. L. Gaiter (Eds.), *Infant stress under intensive care* (pp. 199–226). Baltimore: University Park Press.

Perehudoff, B. (1990). Parents' perceptions of environmental stressors in the special care nursery. *Neonatal Network, 9*, 39–44.

Peters, K. L. (1992). Does routine nursing care complicate the physiologic status of the premature infant with respiratory distress syndrome? *Journal of Perinatal Neonatal Nursing, 6*, 67–84.

Rothchild, B. T., (1966). Incubator isolation as a possible continuing factor to the high incidence of emotional disturbance among premature born persons. *Journal of Genetic Psychology, 110*, 287–304.

Sheldon, S. H., & Bell, E. (1987). Light, sleep and development. *Pediatrics, 79*, 1053.

Shogan, M. G., & Schumann, L. L. (1993). The effect of environmental lighting on the oxygen saturation of preterm infants in the NICU. *Neonatal Network, 12*, 7–13.

Strauch, C., Brandt, S., & Edwards-Beckett, J. (1993). Implementation of a quiet hour: Effect on noise levels and infant sleep states. *Neonatal Network, 12*, 31-35.

Thomas, K. (1989). How the NICU environment sounds to a preterm infant. MCN: *The American Journal of Maternal / Child Nursing, 14*, 249–251.

VandenBerg, K. (1985). Revising the traditional model: An individualized approach to developmental interventions in the intensive care nursery. *Neonatal Network 3*, 32–38.

VandenBerg, K. A. (1990). Behaviorally supportive care for the extremely premature infant. In L. P. Gunderson & C. Kenner (Eds.), *Care of the 24–25 week gestational age infant: Small baby protocol* (pp. 129–157). Petaluma, CA: Neonatal Network.

VandenBerg, K., Gorski, P., & Brazelton, T. B. (1988, November). *Sources of resistance to supporting developmental care and implementing change in the NICU.* Paper presented at the National Conference for Developmental Interventions in Neonatal Care, San Diego, California.

Velasco-Whetsell, M., Evans, J. C., & Wang, M. S. (1992). Do postsuctioning transcutaneous PO2 values change when a neonate's movements are restrained? *Journal of Perinatalogy, 12,* 333–337.

Weibley, T. T. (1989). Inside the incubator. *Maternal-Child Nursing, 14,* 96–100.

Wolke, D. (1987). Environmental and developmental neonatology. *Journal of Reproductive and Infant Psychology, 5,* 17–42.

Zahr, L. (1994). Premature infant responses to noise control by earmuffs: Effects on behavioral and physiologic measures. *Infant Behavior and Development, 17,* 1031.

M. VIRGINIA WYLY ■
SUSAN M. PFALZER, ■
MARY R. SPETH ■

■ CHAPTER 4

Neurobehavioral Development and Support

From the most ancient subject we shall produce the newest science.
Herman Ebbinghaus

■ INTRODUCTION

All infants communicate through their behavior. Sensitive caregivers learn to read these behaviors so that they know when a baby is tired, hungry, or wants to interact. Infants offer cues to how they feel and what they need through their facial expression, body movement, state of consciousness, breathing rate, gestures, and muscle tone.

Full-term infants are born ready to begin interactions with their caregivers. They are remarkably well organized (Fogel, 1990). They use clear signals to communicate with their caregivers. Most full-term newborns are able to quiet themselves. Their states of consciousness are usually clear and easily recognized. They are able to integrate their movements to respond to stimuli. Underlying these behaviors is neurobehavioral organization.

Neurobehavioral organization is governed by the central nervous system functioning and the maturational level of infants. Neurobehavioral organization is the infant's ability to maintain and manage the separate but independent subsystems of physiologic stability, motor, behavioral state, attentional-interaction, and self-regulation in interactions with the environment. Infants' interactions with the environment, their signals, and communicative behaviors are a function of the neurobehavioral organization (Als & Duffy, 1989). At the same time, the interactions impact on the neurobehavioral pattern of organization.

Premature infants, particularly young very low birthweight (VLBW) infants have an immature central nervous system. Consequently, they differ markedly from full-term infants in their capacity to respond to their environment. High-risk infants in neonatal intensive care units do not respond to interactions or changes in the environment like healthy, full-term infants. Depending on their gestational age, birthweight, and medical status they often have a lower threshold for sensory input than do more stable infants. Their behavioral cues are more difficult to read. They show signs of physiologic instability as they attempt to cope with the environmental stimuli. NICU caregivers must modify their care to support the well-being of these high-risk infants (Gorski, 1991).

In this chapter we will examine the neurobehavioral development of premature infants. Neurobehavioral assessment will be reviewed along with the theoretical rationale for providing developmentally supportive care. Implications for developmental care and for the infant and family will be described.

■ NEUROBEHAVIORAL DEVELOPMENT OF PREMATURE INFANTS

Sensitive NICU caregivers must use an infant intervention approach that individualizes care based on each infant's responses to environmental events. Based on the model of subsystems emerging, previously described, caregivers can carefully evaluate infants to determine the current level of organization, stress signs, self-regulatory cues, behavioral capacities, and the appropriate behavioral interventions to use to stabilize and promote the infant's development (Lefrak-Okikawa & Lund, 1993).

VandenBerg (1985) points out that caregivers in the neonatal unit must apply intervention activities to match infants' developmental and medical status. Premature infants face qualitatively different experiences in the hospital than full-term infants. Further, their systems development are different than that of full-term infants. Thus, it is important to understand the course of preterm infant development in order to facilitate the development of these high-risk infants. Let us review some behaviors expected at specific gestational ages (Yecco, 1993). Keep in mind that the medical and physiologic status of the infant can alter the timing and appearance of these behaviors.

Less Than 30 Weeks Gestational Age

Premature infants born less than 30 weeks gestational age may show the following:

- Asymmetric movements of trunk, arms, and legs.
- Flaccid muscle tone, jerky movements.
- Total movements are random.
- Generalized hypotonia.
- Limited resistance to passive range of motion.
- Head lag.
- State behaviors are not well differentiated with sleep states predominating. Active limb movement and rapid eye movement are evident in sleep. Drowsy and alert states are transient if present at all.
- Irregular breathing, including respiratory pauses and gasping.
- Infant unable to coordinate suck and swallow reflexes.
- Startle and reflex smiling are present.
- Eyes open occasionally, eye opening increases toward 30 weeks.
- Visual, kinesthetic, and auditory stimulation may overtax infant resulting in physiological distress.
- Eye movements are rapid and change from one point to another.
- Poor visual acuity; not able to fixate long on human face.
- Hearing is fairly well-developed by 30 weeks.

30 to 32 Weeks Gestational Age

Premature infants between 30 to 32 weeks gestational age may show the following:

- Muscle tone increases.
- Some flexion and coordinated movements are evident.
- State behaviors are more distinctive. Quiet sleep state increases. Some increase in alert and drowsy states.
- Able to focus on visual stimuli.
- Quiets when attending to sound or visual stimuli.
- Quiet sleep increases while active sleep decreases.
- Smoother motor movements but some tremors.
- Hearing is well developed.
- Reflexive smile is evident.
- More resistance to passive movement.
- Brief periods of hand-to-mouth activity.

33 to 36 Weeks Gestational Age

Premature infants between 33 to 36 weeks gestational age may show the following:

■ State behaviors are more clearly defined. Active and quiet sleep alternate regularly with more time spent in active sleep. Can be aroused to an alert state but the stimulation may overtax infant. Increases in crying state.

■ Some coordination of sucking, swallowing, and breathing.

■ Weak muscle tone with some beginnings of head control and leg and trunk support.

■ Reflexes are weak or absent.

■ Infant may briefly respond to auditory or visual stimuli but may become overtaxed and show signs of stress.

■ Evidence of some self-comforting behaviors such as foot clasping or hand-to-mouth maneuvers.

■ Can be consoled by containment or swaddling.

■ Onset of coordination of swallowing, sucking, and breathing.

■ Movements more coordinated, less random.

■ Visually follows and tracks stimuli in a horizontal plane.

■ More resistance to passive movement.

■ Spontaneously flexes and extends limbs.

37 to 40 Weeks Gestational Age

Between 37 to 40 weeks gestational age, premature infants may show the following:

■ Muscle tone increase. Flexion is evident.

■ When placed in an upright position, may support self.

■ Movements coordinated.

■ Can visually track horizontally and vertically.

■ More resistant to passive movement.

■ Primary reflexes, for example, suck and rooting are consistent.

■ Has sleep-wake cycles but not as consistent as full-term infants.

■ Clear, distinct state behaviors. Stays predominately in quiet sleep approximating full-term infant sleep behavior.

■ Visually fixates on the human face and other objects. May show visual preference for stimuli.

■ Alert to sound.

The organization of premature infants' behavioral responses and behavioral competence has been described as occurring in stages (Lott, 1989; Tronick, Scalon, & Scalon, 1987). The following stages have been described:

Stage 1. Inturning: In this stage, the infant attempts to maintain physiologic stability. Energy is directed at doing this, consequently infants are not able to sustain interaction with the environment.

Stage 2. Coming Out: During this stage, premature infants have more physiologic integrity. They are better able to manage changes in environmental stimuli. This stage marks the beginning of interactions with caregivers.

Stage 3. Reciprocating: Preterm infants in this stage are more capable of interactions with caregivers because they are more stable. They can regulate states and give clearer nonverbal cues to their caregivers.

The progression through these stages will depend on the infants' medical condition, gestational age, and physiologic states. Individual infants will be differentially influenced by their environmental interactions. Caregivers must be sensitive to and respond appropriately to each infants' cues.

■ SYNACTIVE THEORY OF DEVELOPMENT

Als' Synactive Theory of Infant Development (1982a) provides a framework for understanding the development of behaviors seen in premature infants. It is also a useful assessment for premature infants as a guide for planning medical and nursing interventions as well as appropriate social interactions with the infant.

Als' synactive theory views the premature infant as an organism ideally suited to intrauterine life who must make dramatic adaptations to the NICU environment to survive. Survival depends on the infant's ability to stabilize and grow in the extrauterine environment. This theoretical model identifies five distinct subsystems within the infant:

1. Physiological or autonomic system
2. Motor system
3. State organizational system
4. Attentional-interactional system
5. Self-regulatory system

In full-term infants these subsystems dynamically interact and support each other reflecting a well-organized, mature nervous system. Full-term infants have no difficulty negotiating the environment because a stable autonomic and motor system allows the infant to control state behaviors, self-regulate their stress responses to the environment, and remain available for interaction with caregivers. Premature infants, depending on their gestational age and neurological maturation, will have varying degrees of emergence of these subsystems.

Physiologic or autonomic stability is an absolute prerequisite for the emergence of the other subsystems. Without it there can be no state regulation. Stressors in the NICU environment, for example, suctioning, bright lights, and heel sticks can cause profound disequilibrium particularly in very fragile infants. Distinct states of consciousness such as quiet alert, active alert, active sleep, quiet sleep, crying, and drowsy are easily identified in full-term infants but not in immature premature infants. States in premature infants are transitory if present at all. As premature infants develop, their behavioral states emerge and become more robust. Interaction with caregivers will occur as the infant's nervous system matures and the subsystems function adaptively.

To better understand the challenges facing premature infants in the NICU, Als' subsystems will be examined in more detail. The behaviors of premature infants that represent the level of function in each subsystem will be identified. Keep in mind that although the importance of identifying intrasubsystem function, is just as important as identifying the relationship and supportive interplay between subsystems.

Als (1982b) describes this subsystem as the observable strategies the infant uses to maintain equilibrium between the subsystems that are currently in play. Even extremely premature infants can self-regulate by completely tuning out the environment. With neurodevelopmental maturity, self-regulation techniques become much more sophisticated. Self-regulation is the "glue" that holds the subsystems together, allowing the infant to effectively utilize all of the subsystems. Each subsystem is described in this section.

Physiological System

The physiological or autonomic subsystem is the first system to emerge. For very young infants, for example, 24–32 weeks, their behavioral cues are primarily physiological. The physiological system encompasses infants' bodily functions including heart rate; breathing behavior; skin color; autonomic mediated movements such as tremors, startles, twitching, eye floating, and eye rolling; and digestive functions such as vomiting, hiccoughs, gagging, and bowel movements. The occurrence and intensity of each of these functions is a clue to how well infants are responding to the environment.

Heart Rate

Premature infants have a more rapid heart rate than older children or adults. A regular, smooth heart rate indicates the infant is stable; however irregularities in heart rate are not uncommon in premature infants. Environmental events such as medical interventions, feeding or diapering may affect heart rate. In response to environmental stressors, premature infants may have bradycardia, a decrease in heart rate below 80 beats per minute or tachycardia which is rapid heart rate over 180 beats per minute.

Respiration

Smooth, regular respiration is a behavioral indication that the infant is stable. Respiratory irregularity or other respiratory cues such as tachypnea or rapid breathing, apneic episodes, and labored breathing are signs of problems or medical difficulties. In fragile or young premature infants, respiratory irregularities will occur in response to environmental stimuli.

Skin Color

Mild color changes are common in premature infants. It is important to assess baseline changes that normally occur in infants in order to assess significant color changes. Common color changes that indicate distress are dusky color of face, body, and limbs; pale nose and fingertips; and mottled appearance of face and body.

Thus, an infant who is distressed could be assessed physiologically by observing body twitching, cessation of breathing, increased gastric residuals, bowel movement straining, color change, and tachypnea. Throughout the infant's stay in the NICU, these systems must function. If they do not function efficiently, the infant will die. During particularly stressful times or when the infant is very ill, there will be a noticeable deterioration in the infant's ability to maintain basic bodily functions. The emergence of functioning of the other subsytems are dependent on stability within this system.

Autonomic Mediated Movements

Spontaneous startle responses often seen in very young premature infants indicate central nervous system immaturity. Severe startles may indicate the infant is distressed. Excessive twitches and tremors are more common in very young preterm infants; in older infants these abrupt body movements can be a sign of neurological immaturity. Another sign of CNS immaturity is eye floating. This occurs when the infant's eyes appear to float up and are not focused. All of these signs may occur in response to overstimulation.

Digestive Signs

Spitting up, gagging, hiccoughing, and bowel straining can be signs of distress. These behaviors may also occur normally, so it is important to assess the context in which they occur. For example, they might appear after vital signs or a medical procedure and would probably be signs of stress.

Motor System

Infants' ability to move and position their body is a gradually emerging activity. Very early premature infants have few purposeful movements of arms and legs. Twitching, jerky limb movements are typical in young premature infants. It is very difficult for them to overcome the pull of gravity. Poor energy and diminished muscle tone make movements that do occur very weak.

As infants grow and mature, they will replace the generally limp, flaccid postures of prematurity with the flexion and increased muscle tone characteristic of full-term infants. Infants begin to withdraw from painful stimuli as they mature, no longer passive and accepting of interventions. Jittery, nonpurposeful movement will eventually be replaced by smooth, purposeful movements of arms and legs. The intrauterine environment provides the flexion, containment, and midline positioning that is normal for developing infants; if born prematurely, the components of proper positioning and containment must be provided by the caregiver so that proper muscle tone and development of movement patterns can be normalized. Poor positioning can cause an enormous amount of energy loss as infants will often seek a position of comfort. This energy is much better conserved for growth.

State Organizational System

Infant states are organized in distinct patterns of physical and physiological responses of rest and arousal (Fogel, 1991). It is the infant's way of exerting control over the type of interaction he receives from the environment. Understanding the infant's state is important because it provides signals that cue caregivers as to the infant's readiness to interact or his need to be left alone.

Infants' state behavior is determined by a constellation of observable behaviors including facial expression, body movements, eye movements or eye opening, respiration, and muscle tone or movements.

The first emerging two states are the sleep states. Quiet sleep (State 1) is characterized by regular respiration, very few body movements, and deep sleep. This sleep state develops with maturity. Active sleep (State 2) is observed in younger premature infants (less than 30 weeks of gestation). They experience rapid eye movements; irregular, primarily abdominal, respiration; and some body movements. State 3, drowsy, represents a transitional state between asleep and awake states. An infant's eyes may be open or closed—if open, they have a glassy look. The infant exhibits facial grimacing, variable motor activity, fluttering eyelids, and irregular respirations. States 4, 5, and 6 are the awake states. In the quiet alert state (State 4) the infant moves about minimally and can focus alertly on a source of stimulation. In this state, respirations are regular and eyes are bright and shiny. It is in this state that infants may be able to look at their caregivers. As infants enter the active awake state (State 5), their movements increase with increasing fussiness and irritability. The crying state (State 6) is indicated by intense, rhythmic crying accompanied by increased motor movements.

Unlike their full-term counterparts, premature infants have a limited repertoire of conscious states. In addition, very young premature infants move quickly between states, which makes diagnosis difficult. These infants sleep restlessly most of the time and have only fleeting moments of alertness. They seem to be oblivious to their environment and may not even react to painful interventions. Crying is absent, and a weak facial grimace may be the only observable reaction. In the NICU this situation can be very dangerous because, in a crisis situation, these infants will quickly decompensate physiologically with very little warning.

Alert states that enable social interaction are extremely rare in preterm infants. As premature infants mature, they have regular occurrences of the active alert state. Caregivers can watch for those infant behaviors that indicate a readiness to interact, for example, eyes opening in response to touch or auditory stimulation; regular respirations; and no, or controlled, body movements. In premature infants, however, the active alert state can be easily disrupted. If an interaction becomes too stressful, premature infants may try to look away or become hyper-alert. Frantic motor movements and crying may follow. If the stressor continues, this behavior can deteriorate and result in physiologic decompensation. They may develop apnea, lack of breathing, with a concomitant decrease in heart rate that can be life threatening.

As infants get older, they remain in each state for a longer period of time and will make state transitions more predictably.

Attentional Interactive System

The attentional/interactive system refers to the quality of infants' alert state. It is the ability of infants to attend to and interact with people and objects in their environment.

Als (1982a) refers to this subsystem as the essence of humanness. In her view, the survival of the human species depends on the ability to attend to and interact with others. Certainly, parents are very anxious for their infants to begin opening their eyes and interacting with them. Even with very sick infants, parents may encourage them to try to open their eyes. Unfortunately, this capacity is dependant on the maturation and stability of the autonomic, motor, and state subsystems that precede it. So, parents may be disappointed when their infant is unresponsive. It takes a knowledgeable and patient parent to wait for and identify the quiet alert state that signals the infants' readiness to interact. Further vigilance is required to assure that these early and brief periods of alertness are not overexploited, tiring the infant and causing dangerous stress responses.

Self-Regulatory System

This subsystem represents the ability of infants to utilize physiologic, motor, and state strategies to independently manage environmental stimulation and self-organization. Successful self-regulation allows infants to maintain stability by protecting themselves from stressors. Some of these "self-regulatory" behaviors include bringing hand-to-mouth, sucking, grasping, hand clasping, and/or postural change. A high level of neurobehavioral maturity has been achieved when an infant successfully manages environmental stress without physiologically decompensating (Als, 1982b; Als et al., 1986).

Als' synactive theory of infant development provides a framework through which caregivers and parents understand the behaviors they see in premature infants. By simply looking at infants and assessing signs and behaviors, caregivers can provide what the infant needs in the least stressful manner. This is the basis of developmentally supportive care. Identifying behaviors that indicate the level of functioning in each subsystem supporting the infant as the subsystems mature and stabilize prepares the foundation for later developing subsystems and optimizes the neurobehavioral development of premature infants.

Using Als' framework to assess infants and plan interventions, medical staff can provide care in developmentally supportive ways (Hiniker & Moreno, 1994). The goal is to carefully observe infants, assess their behavioral stability, and then provide appropriate interventions. Staff can assist parents to observe their infant's behaviors and reactions. This process must begin as early as possible to involve parents in developmentally supported care. Field (1987) notes that broadening the knowledge, skill, and experience of parents not only enhances infant development, but also improves parenting skills.

As infants grow and mature in the NICU, what constitutes developmentally supportive care changes. In the beginning, or the acute stage, the primary focus of medical staff and parents is survival. The rule of the NICU is usually to provide aggressive interventions utilizing all the available technology. Often, little thought is given to developmental support. The priority of sustaining life for very premature sick infants is a never ending flow of disruptive, sometimes painful medical and nursing procedures. Time for uninterrupted rest or positive touching interaction is often not considered a priority.

The acute stage ends as infants stabilize. Many infants are then considered healthy, growing premature babies. A good number of them, however, will become chronically ill. As infants move from acute to chronic illness, developmental needs change as well as medical and nursing approaches. The developmental care needs of acute and chronic care infants are necessarily different because growth and maturation require more attention to environmental input. In chronic care, many of the earlier, aggressive interventions are no longer necessary because the infant has now developed relatively stable physiologic functioning. Energy is now devoted to growth and development. Unfortunately, many of these chronic infants will remain in the acute care setting because many hospitals do not have transitional care units or the infants are still too unstable to be moved. Chronic infants challenge medical and nursing staff to provide care appropriate to each infant's developmental level. This requires ongoing assessment and planning.

■ NEUROBEHAVIORAL ASSESSMENT

Assessment of premature infants can be done by neonatal nurses, physicians, educators, and therapists. Neurobehavioral assessments provide information about the infant's behavioral organization and stability. There are several reasons for doing assessments. Assessments are used to design care for individual infants in the NICU (Tribotti & Stein, 1992). They can be used to determine an infant's tolerance for interactions in family visits or during procedures. Assessments also are used to measure infants' progress during hospitalization (Merenstein, 1994).

Before undertaking an assessment, NICU care providers must consider several things. How intrusive is the assessment process? Because of premature infants' limited tolerance of handling or sensory input, the examiner must determine whether the assessment process itself will tax the infant. If the assessment involves touching or moving the infant it may cause undue stress for the infant. Simply handling a fragile premature infant may create instability (American Occupational Therapy Association, 1993). The examiner must ask whether the timing of the assessment process is appropriate for the infant. The examiner should be clear about the purpose of the assessment. Why is it being done? What will be learned or changed as a result of the information gathered? Finally, examiners must consider their role as they plan assessments. During these assessments, the examiner interacts with the infant and becomes a part of the infant's social milieu.

Several assessments have been developed for assessment of preterm behavior. Some of the assessments require certification. The certification process involves an initial introduction to the test and then observation of the trainee using the assessment procedures. The trainee must complete required reading and practice and then successfully complete a required reliability in administering and scoring the assessment.

Neonatal Behavioral Assessment Scale (NBAS)

The Neonatal Behavioral Assessment Scale measures the interactions and behavioral organization of full-term newborns (Brazelton,1973, 1984). This assessment (NBAS) is the template for the APIB designed by Als for premature infants. The NBAS incorporates an approach that reflects current knowledge of the rich behavioral repertoire of newborn infants. A major construct is the importance of state and arousal in the infant's ability to regulate environmental stimuli. The state of the infant is manipulated while observing the infant's capacity to process environmental events.

A basic tenet of the NBAS is that neonates are active rather than passive beings who interact with their environment. The behavioral range of test items assess the neonate's ability to respond to social and nonsocial stimuli, to habituate, to self-organize, and control motor activity and states. The examiner maneuvers the newborn from the sleep to awake state and notes the state robustness, state changes, and the ways that specific environmental responses occur within states. These are considered valid indicators of overall neurological functioning.

A unique feature of the NBAS is that the examiner attempts to elicit the infant's best performance rather than an average performance score. This means that the examiners must know how to handle newborns to obtain optimal performance.

Assessment of Preterm Infant Behavior (APIB)

The APIB is designed to assess the five subsystems identified in Als' Synactive Theory (physiologic, motoric, state system, attentional-interactional, self-regulation) before, during, and following environmental maneuvers (Als & Duffy, 1989). The infant's current level of functioning is assessed through these maneuvers. The examiner de-

termines how well the infant adapts to these maneuvers and the toleration level of the infant for the input of stimuli. The infant's behavioral organization and disorganization is assessed by applying increasingly demanding environmental stimuli.

Signs of stability and instability are assessed in each subsystem
(Als, 1982a). The signs in each of the areas are:

	Stability Signs	**Instability Signs**
Motoric	■ Smooth coordinated movements ■ Good tone ■ Able to use motor strategies, for example, hand-to-mouth maneuvers ■ Foot/hand clasping	■ Diffuse motoric activity ■ Hypertonicity ■ Hypotonic/Flaccid ■ Jerky motion
Physiologic	■ Regular respirations ■ Stable color ■ Stable digestion	■ Irregular respiration ■ Color changes ■ Digestive problems, for example, gagging, spitting up, hiccoughing
State	■ Clear states ■ Robust state behaviors ■ Self-calming behaviors ■ Maintains periods of quiet alert states	■ Diffuse states ■ Transition states predominate ■ State behaviors diffuse and change rapidly
Attentional/ Interactional	■ Visually attends to stimuli ■ Quiets body movements to stimuli ■ Attends to auditory stimuli	■ Gaze aversion ■ Fussiness ■ Shows physiologic ■ instability to auditory/ visual input

Naturalistic Observations of Newborn Behavior (NONB)

The NONB is an assessment of infants who are unable to tolerate
handling or touch (Als, 1984). The assessment uses the synactive theory framework. The infant is observed before, during, and after caregiving procedures. Through systematic observations the examiner assesses the infant's levels of stability, instability, and self-regulation
capabilities. Measures of physiologic functioning, for example, respiration, heart rate, and oxygen saturation, are charted. Based on the
assessment results, specific care recommendations including modifi-
cations of the infant's environment.

Neurobehavioral Assessment of the Preterm Infant (NAPI)

The Neurobehavioral Assessment of the Preterm Infant is designed to measure preterm infants' level of functioning (Korner & Thom, 1990). The test assesses premature infants from 32 weeks gestational age to full term. Test items assess motor development and activity, orientation to animate and inanimate visual and auditory stimuli, behavioral states, and range of passage movements. Some test items have been adapted from the Brazelton (1973) *Neonatal Behavioral Assessment Scale*. Like the Brazelton assessment, the examiner attempts to get best performance from the infant through repeated observations. Much of the test consists of observing infant behaviors, rather than handling the infant.

Conclusion

The assessment process provides an in-depth look at the neurobehavioral organization of preterm infants. Through careful observations the infant's interactions with the environment and toleration of environmental input can be determined. Family members can be included in the assessment by providing information about their infant's responses or consulting on care plans. Assessments can serve as a teaching tool to assist staff and parents to understand the cues and behaviors of the infant in order to modify their interactional styles and interact more effectively.

The care that high-risk infants receive in NICUs has recently come under close scrutiny (Creger, 1989). NICU caregivers must deliver care in such a way to not only keep infants alive, but also protect them from potential threats to normal growth and development. This approach to care in NICUs is known as developmentally supportive care.

Developmentally supportive care should begin when the infant enters the intensive care nursery. Such care requires NICU health providers to assess each infant's developmental level as well as the level of medical acuity within the context of providing medical interventions (Miller & Quinn-Hurst, 1994). An assessment allows NICU caregivers to individualize their care, recognize signs of self-regulation and stress, and use these signs to promote infant stability. Signs of stress mean that the infant is overtaxed, tired, or disorganized. These signs communicate to NICU caregivers that the infant needs time out, the environment is overstimulating, or that medical interventions should stop if possible. Signs of self-regulation communicate that the infant is stable, organized, and has some self-control. When infants show signs of stability and are alert, then social interactions are more often possible.

NICU caregivers can use their assessment of neurobehavioral development to plan care. Developmental care can be implemented whether infants are seriously ill and require acute care or have stabilized and need chronic care. Prior to developmental interventions, the infant should be carefully observed and behaviors documented. The following questions should be answered before starting developmental care interventions:

- In what situations does the infant function well?
- What helps the infant to function smoothly?
- What medical/caregiving procedures upset the infant?
- What positions does the infant tolerate?
- What positions agitate the infant?
- What are the infant's time-out cues?
- If the infant shows signs of stress, how long does the stress last?
- How much handling does the infant experience daily?
- What is the amount of handling the infant can tolerate?
- What does the infant do to calm herself?
- What support does the infant need to be calmed or consoled?
- What caregiving interventions are effective in assisting the infant to organize and self-regulate?

■ ACUTE AND CHRONIC CARE

Acute Care

Technological advances in the care of high-risk neonates are truly remarkable, and with these advances mortality rates continue to drop. It is now possible to save infants as early as 24 weeks of gestation. It is essential that professionals working in the NICU use means at their disposal to ensure not only survival, but a high quality of life for these very vulnerable infants and their families. As NICU health professionals address medical needs of these vulnerable infants so too should they respond to infants' developmental and psychosocial needs. The long-term developmental outcome of premature infants is influenced by their interactions with their caregivers and their environments.

This is often a difficult task, since premature infants may spend enormous amounts of time in the NICU. An infant born at 24 weeks of gestation, for example, will spend a minimum of 16 weeks in the NICU if all goes well. The length of stay can dramatically increase if the infant succumbs to one or more of the many possible complications. Not only do premature infants experience many medical procedures, but the hospital environment provides a very different sensory input than the home (High & Gorski, 1985).

When they first enter the NICU, infants are often acutely ill. The primary focus of parents and health care team is survival. During the acute phase of illness, an infant is handled often. As a result of excessive handling, these fragile infants may respond negatively to any touch. Studies done in NICUs have found that infants are handled in ranges of 60 to 234 times per 24 hours (Graven et al., 1992). This contact was mostly caregiving, defined as handling during medical and nursing procedures. As the acute phase passed and recovery took place, contact became much more social but not always contingent on infant's behavior.

Many clinicians agree that the best approach to acute care is the "Minimal Stimulation" protocol. Many nurseries are coming to realize the benefit of this hands off approach to care. By using monitoring equipment to observe physiologic signs and handling the infant only when absolutely necessary, stressful events are kept to a minimum, and precious energy is conserved for growth (Peters, 1992). Every routine intervention should be carefully considered for its risk and potential benefit to the infant. When necessary procedures are performed, evaluate the infant's response and provide support as needed. For example, painful procedures may require administration of analgesics beforehand (Johnston & Stevens, 1990; Lawson, 1988). Increased oxygen and frequent rest periods may be needed, with physical support in the form of containment and proper positioning. Staff may reduce excessive noise and light to minimize environmental stimulation.

Periods of uninterrupted sleep are essential for neonates' healthy growth and development. Full-term infants sleep for 20 or more hours a day, and premature infants sleep even more; growth hormones like Cortisol are more active during periods of sleep. Thus sleep promotes growth in premature infants. Sleep deprivation in adult ICU patients has been well documented and can cause profound disorientation, a state referred to as ICU "psychosis." Similarly, investigators are concerned about sleep interruption in fragile premature infants who are handled frequently.

Utilizing the five assessment areas described by Als (1982a) (Autonomic, Motoric, Behavioral State, Attentional Interaction, and Self-Regulation) individualized developmentally supportive care, based on an ongoing assessment of the infant's responses to interventions can be planned (Becker, Grunwald, Moorman, & Stuhr, 1991). It is a widely held belief that this approach to NICU care has the potential to avoid behavioral and physiological disorganization and thus enhance the normal development of the infant (Als, Lester, Tronick, & Brazelton, 1982; Yecco, 1993).

Case Study

Let us look at a case example of an infant in the acute phase admitted to a large NICU at 24 weeks of gestation. Necessary medical interventions will be described and suggestions for assuring they are developmentally supportive will be given within the context of Al's five assessment areas.

> D.J. is an 866 gram (1 lb. 14 oz.) 24-week white male born in a community hospital to a 24-year-old primigravida. He was picked up by a transport nurse and taken to a 54 bed Level III Neonatal Intensive Care Unit in a nearby city. On admission, he was noted to be a very small frail infant with gelatinous skin and fused eyelids. D.J. was critically ill and required maximum ventilatory support. All his physiological needs that were met by the placental maternal unit were provided by the medical team.

Autonomic

Physiologically, D.J. is in a very immature state. Without a ventilator breathing for him, he would quickly die. His heart will continue to beat only as long as his breathing is supported artificially. Indeed bradycardia, or a sudden decrease in heart rate, is one of the first indications that the environment is becoming too stressful. His nutritional needs must be met by intravenous routes because his digestive system is unable to accept food. All of D.J.'s body systems are functioning minimally, and all of his energy is devoted to simply staying alive.

D. J. will require extensive medical interventions such as endotracheal intubation, IV insertion, arterial line placement, suctioning, diagnostic procedures, blood drawing, weighing, vital sign assessment, and ongoing physical/neurological assessment.

Motor System

As D.J. lies on the warming table, it is obvious that he has very little motoric control. The flexor tone seen in full-term infants is absent. He stays in whatever position the caregiver leaves him in. There is no energy to find a position of comfort so he must be assisted by a caregiver. The model for positioning is the position experienced during intrauterine life. Flexion, containment, and midline positioning of extremities is the goal.

Infants in the NICU are usually positioned in three main positions. Prone is the most therapeutic and utilizes gravity to aid respiration. Side-lying entails placing the infant on either right or left side. One advantage to this position is that limb flexion and hand-to-mouth maneuvers are possible with positioning aids. Supine is the least desirable because it promotes extension and allows for the gravitational pull on thoracic muscles and extremities. By using positioning aids, professionals can properly provide motoric support and environmental positioning support for these fragile infants.

State System

During the acute phase in very early premature infants, there is relatively little state differentiation. Of the six infant states quiet sleep, active sleep, drowsy, quiet alert, active awake, and crying (Wyly & Allen, 1990), sick premature infants experience sleep states and very brief alert times. In fact, the ability to shut down and avoid interaction is necessary to provide time for healing and is probably one of the premature infant's greatest strengths (Yecco, 1993).

Caregivers must learn to watch babies and identify states. Sleep states must never be interrupted unless absolutely necessary. Routine nursing care activities should be altered to take into account behavioral cues of infants. Parents need to understand the inability of the infant at this early stage to maintain alertness. If they are told this is normal behavior and temporary, most parents will not continue with inappropriate stimulation in an effort to wake the infant up. Gorski, (1985), states that the result of teaching parents about unique premature infant behaviors is that they will be able to identify behavioral stages of infant recovery. In this way parents can come to appreciate the infant's progress even though their infant is not able to show expected full-term behaviors.

Attentional System

Clearly, D.J. is totally unable to take in cognitive social and emotional information from the environment in the acute stage. He is a purely physiologic being using every ounce of energy to stay alive. As he recovers and matures, this ability will emerge. By about 28 weeks of gestation, he will have greater alertness and awareness of his environment. Behavioral responses, if carefully elicited, may be seen briefly (Borland, 1989). Likewise, self-regulatory behaviors are nonexistent. It will be a long time before D.J. will have the sophistication or central nervous system integrity to pick and choose what stimuli in the environment he will attend to and which he will not. Until then, he is at the mercy of the potentially stressful NICU and will need the help of his allies, the medical team and his parents.

Chronic Care

As time passes, the medical and nursing care becomes less technical and invasive. Indirect monitoring of physiologic status is the rule and less physical manipulation of the infant is required. The focus of the medical team now is to maximize growth and prepare the infant and parents for discharge. Progress during this growth period is very slow with potential crises and setbacks. About with infection or feeding difficulties can be a major setback and significantly increase length of stay.

Some infants do not progress as well as others and may develop chronic health problems like bronchopulmonary dysplasia, a very serious lung disease that at worst causes death and at the least prolongs hospital stay and delays normal growth and development. In many NICUs, these infants are referred to as "chronics." Clearly, the sheer length of time that infants spend in the stressful environment of the NICU points up the need to modify that environment for support of infants and families.

The medical care, nursing care, and parent involvement during the acute phase of illness differ markedly from that of the chronic phase. The common thread that underlies chronic care is a focus on doing what needs to be done in a developmentally supportive way so that adverse effects of intrusive medical/nursing care will be minimized and the integrity of the growing, developing infant is preserved and enhanced.

Three months later, D.J. is now 36 weeks gestation, almost full term. He weighs about 4½ pounds, has been off the respirator for only a few weeks, and requires supplemental oxygen. Physiologic stability has been achieved, and social behaviors are emerging. Feeding by bottle has just started but is not going well because D.J. has very significant lung disease, and eating requires too much energy. Medications designed to ease breathing have the unwanted side effect of irritability. Very often it is difficult to identify causes of the almost ceaseless crying when D.J. is awake. Monitoring is less invasive now and medical interventions much less frequent. Social interactions and caregiving tasks are more normalized; D.J. can be held and rocked now, allowing his mother the opportunity to provide more natural mothering activities.

Unfortunately, D.J.'s extremely premature birth has left his lungs so damaged he must remain in the acute care setting of the NICU even though he is now chronically ill. Progress will be very slow. Plans are being made to send him home and to prepare his parents for his discharge to their care. Even if he goes home, it will be about 2 years before his lungs will recover, and he still is at very high risk of dying from lung disease.

The care of chronic care infants represents a challenge to families and NICU health professionals. These infants must cope with an environment that is inconsistent and does not often offer contingent stimulation so typical of full-term infants in the home environment. Care for chronic infants in the NICU encompasses both medical interventions and developmentally appropriate methods that foster growth and development. While very young, fragile infants in acute care cannot tolerate stimulation, older infants may be capable of responding to one or multimodal stimuli. For infants who must spend several months or years in the hospital, health care professionals must create developmentally appropriate methods that match the infants' special needs (Wells, DeBoard-Burns, Cook, & Mitchell, 1994).

Now let us turn our attention to D.J., using Als' subsystems as an assessment guide. As D.J. approaches full term, he in some ways resembles a full-term newborn but, in most ways, does not. Because of his illness and long stay in the hostile environment of the NICU, he is behaviorally very different from a full-term infant. In terms of Als' assessment categories he has nevertheless come a long way. Physiologically, D.J. has matured. His heart rate is steady and rarely drops even if he is stressed. Like a full-term infant, he is more likely to have increases in heart rate related to stress. His digestive and excretory functions have matured. If he must work too hard to bottle feed, however, he may vomit. The energy required to feed normally may cause weight loss. Lung damage, caused by many weeks on a respirator, have affected D.J.'s ability to breathe well. If he becomes stressed, his respiratory rate may increase rapidly and he will become cyanotic requiring increased amounts of oxygen. If the stress becomes overwhelming, he may have to go back on the respirator. It is absolutely essential that D.J. be watched very closely for physiological stress signs and that he continue to be protected from stress in the NICU. If these responses are allowed to continue and escalate, the results could be respiratory arrest and death.

Motor System

D.J. is motorically similar to a full-term infant. Flexion is the dominant posture; jitteriness and tremors have disappeared. Arms and legs are stronger now, allowing him to push away noxious stimuli and to vigorously withdraw from painful procedures. In order to perform medical and nursing procedures, it may be necessary to restrain him and will take longer to comfort and settle him afterwards. Like a newborn baby, he will be comforted by holding, hugging, and patting. A pacifier is a welcome source of comfort during stressful interventions. Unlike a normal newborn, when stressed, D.J. will exhibit unusual motoric behaviors such as profound arching of the back, and he will be much more difficult to console or "settle."

State System

Alert periods are emerging. D.J. now spends time quietly awake in his crib, looking at toys or a mobile or his caregivers' faces. Sleep becomes deeper and more peaceful with less movement. The sleep state in premature infants should be respected, and interventions and feeding should be planned for awake times. It is about this time that demand feeding schedules are instituted so that periods of uninterrupted sleep will occur. This approach to care of chronically ill or healthy, growing premature infants conserves energy and encourages the development of natural diurnal and circadian rhythms.

It is now much easier for D.J.'s mother to care for him, and she will gradually take more and more responsibility for his care in preparation for taking him home. From the beginning of his NICU stay, he has recognized his mother's voice and experienced her touch. Her patience is rewarded as D.J. looks into her face, alerts to her voice and relaxes as she holds and comforts him.

Self-Regulation

Although D.J. is older, he has only a limited repertoire of self-regulatory behaviors and will continue to need help in dealing with the extraordinary stress of the NICU, which remains his home. Providing containment with blankets or hands will help him maintain control. Controlling noise, light, and handling remain important components of his care. By developing an Individualized Developmental Care Plan using input from parents, nurses, and other team members, a consistent approach to care will be assured. This consistent approach will help D.J. grow and mature in a more normal way and will maximize his innate ability to handle his world.

■ MANAGING NEONATAL PAIN

Pain management has posed many challenges for NICU health providers. It is in the best interest of the infant to control and prevent pain to promote comfort, decrease stress, and support the healing process. The advent of neurobehavioral assessment has provided a useful vehicle for assessing preterm infants' response to painful stimuli. Observation of infant signs of stress and instability of physiologic functions can guide appropriate pain management interventions. Nurses who are consistently at the infant's bedside can observe changes in the infant's behavior, physiologic stability, and facial expressions (see Figure 4–1). Through their observation skills and attention to changes in the infant's physiologic cues, nurses can act as the infant's "voice" when the infant experiences pain.

There has not always been a voice for vulnerable premature infants who cannot speak for themselves. Historically, painful procedures such as surgery were done without anesthesia and analgesia. Anesthesia, which results in loss of sensation, and analgesia, which causes alleviates pain sensation, were believed to be dangerous to the infant's survival. In fact, the known negative side effects of these drug effects occur rarely (Rogers, 1992). In most medical procedures, safe analgesics are available for even very fragile infants (Bauchner, May, & Coates, 1992).

Until the 1980s it was believed that babies do not experience pain (Berry & Gregory, 1987). Researchers began to investigate behavioral and physiological changes associated with pain. Levine and Gordan (1982) found that infants had different types of cries from pain, discomfort, and hunger. Williamson and Williamson (1983) examined infants' physiological responses such as respirations and heart rate to circumcision with and without anesthesia. Those infants who underwent surgery without anesthesia had physiological changes which the authors interpreted as response to pain. In 1987, Anand and Hickey published a landmark review on the effects of pain

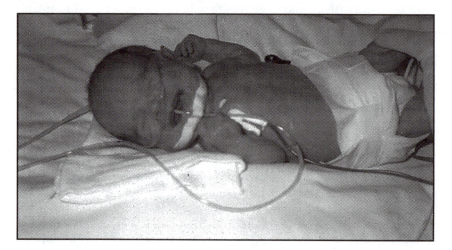

Figure 4–1. Premature infant pain indicated by facial grimace and clenched fist. (Photograph courtesy of Children's Hospital of Buffalo Department of Medical Photography.)

on neonates in the *New England Journal of Medicine*. Their review provided convincing evidence that premature infants and full-term neonates had neural pathways capable of conducting painful stimuli.

Armed with this evidence, NICUs have begun to institute pain protocols to ensure that infants are not allowed to experience pain unnecessarily (Mastropaolo, Consenstein, & Pergolizzi, 1994). These protocols now emphasize assessment of neurobehavioral organization as indicators of pain in addition to information on pain management procedures using drugs and environmental changes.

Staff training on pain management focuses on pain assessment and appropriate interventions. Training includes teaching staff the behavioral indices of pain, for example, changes in facial expression, state changes, bodily movements, vocalizations, and physiological indicators such as increased heart rate, blood pressure changes, changes in levels of oxygen saturation, and color changes (see Figure 4–2). Interventions to reduce pain include protecting the infant from excessive environmental stimulation, modifying the environment, for example, dimming unit lights, covering isolettes, reducing noise, providing containment for the infant, and clustering or spreading out care. Facilitated tucking, which is motoric containment of infant's arms and legs in a flexed, midline position, has been found to attenuate infants' behavioral and physiologic responses to pain (Colditz, 1991;

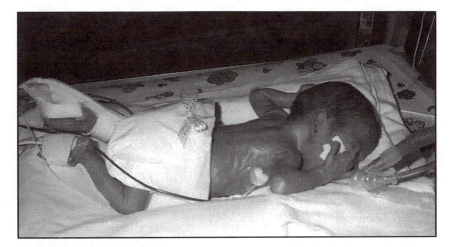

Figure 4–2. Pain in a premature infant can be monitored through physiological indicators such as increased heart rate, blood pressure changes, and changes in oxygen saturation levels. (Photograph courtesy of Children's Hospital of Buffalo Department of Medical Photography.)

Corff, Seideman, Venkataraman, Lutes, & Yates, 1995). The timing and use of analgesics and anesthesia are also part of the pain protocol.

■ **SUMMARY**

Als' synactive theory of development describes infant development in terms of neurobehavioral organization. According to this theory separate subsystems of development interact and affect the overall neurobehavioral organization of the infant. The subsystems are physiologic or autonomic, motoric, state, and attentional/interactional. The infant's behavioral competence is the result of the subsystems' development, integration, and interactions.

Neurobehavioral assessments determine the level of infant competence in interacting with the environment. Several assessments have been developed for premature infants. One such assessment is the Assessment of Premature Infant Behavior (APIB). These assessments utilize infant communication cues and threshold for environmental interactions. NICU caregivers use assessments to plan developmental care that supports preterm infants' development and self-regulatory strategies.

Assessment of neurobehavioral competence is useful in the care of acutely ill preterm infants as well as infants who are more stable or chronic. Planning acute or chronic care requires ongoing assessment of individual infants.

■ **REFERENCES**

Als, H. (1982a). Toward a synactive theory of development: Promise for the assessment and support of infant individuality. *Infant Mental Health Journal, 3*(4), 229–243.

Als, H. (1982b). Manual for the assessment of preterm infants' behavior (APIB). In H. E. Fitzgerald, B. M. Lester, & M. W. Yogman (Eds), *Theory and research in behavioral pediatrics* (Vol. 1, pp. 65–132). New York: Plenum Press.

Als, H. (1984). *Manual for the naturalistic observation of newborn behavior in preterm and fullterm infants*. Boston: Children's Hospital.

Als, H., & Duffy, F. (1989). Neurobehavioral assessment in the newborn period: Opportunity for early detection on later learning disablitites and for early intervention. *Birth Defects, 25*, 127–152.

Als, H., Lawhon, G., Brown, E., Duffy, F., McNulty, G., & Blickman, J. G. (1986). Individualized behavioral and environmental care for the very low birth weight preterm infant at high risk for bronchopulmonary dysplasia: Neonatal intensive care unit and developmental outcome. *Pediatrics, 78*, 1123–1132.

Als, H., Lester, B. M., Tronick, E., & Brazelton, T. B. (1982). Towards a research instrument for the assessment of preterm infants' behavior. In H.

E. Fitzgerald, B. M. Lester & M. W. Yogman (Eds.), *Theory and research in behavioral pediatrics* (Vol 1, pp. 35–63). New York: Plenum Press.

American Occupational Therapy Association. (1993). Knowledge and skills for occupational therapy practice in the neonatal intensive care unit. *The American Journal of Occupational Therapy, 47*, 1100–1105.

Anand, K. J. S., & Hickey, P. B. (1987). Pain and its effect in the human neonate and fetus. *New England Journal of Medicine, 317*, 1121–1132.

Bauchner, H., May, A., & Coates, E. (1992). Use of analgesic agents for invasive medical procedures in pediatrics and neonatal intensive care units. *Journal of Pediatrics, 121*, 647–649.

Becker, P. T., Grunwald, P. C., Moorman, J., & Stuhr, S. (1991). Outcome of developmentally supportive nursery care for very low birthweight infants. *Nursing Research, 40*, 150–155.

Berry, F. A., & Gregory, G. A. (1987). Do premature infants require anesthesia for surgery? *Anesthesiology, 67*, 291–293.

Borland, M. (1989). Neuromotor development in C. J. Semmler (Ed.), *A guide to care and management of the VLBW infant* (pp. 216–232). Tucson, AZ: Therapy Skill Builders.

Brazelton, T. B. (1973). *Neonatal Behavioral Assessment National Spastics Society Monograph*. Philadelphia, PA: J. B. Lippincot.

Brazelton, T. B. (1984). Neonatal Behavioral Assessment (2nd ed.). *Clinics in Developmental Medicine No. 88*. Philadelphia: J. P. Lippincott.

Colditz, P. B. (1991). Review article: Management of pain in the newborn infant. *Journal of Paediatric Child Health, 27*, 11–15.

Corff, K. E., Seideman, R., Venkataraman, P. S., Lutes, L., & Yates, B. (1995). Facilitated tucking: A nonpharmacologic comfort measure for pain in preterm neonates. *Journal of Obstetric, Gynecologic and Neonatal Nursing, 24*, 143–147.

Creger, P. J. (1989). *Developmental interventions for preterm and high risk infants: Self study modules for professionals*. Tucson, AZ: Therapy Skill Builders.

Field, T. (1987). Affective and interactive disturbances in infants. In J. D. Osofsky (Ed.), *Handbook of infant development* (2nd ed.). New York: Wiley.

Fogel, A. (1990). The process of developmental change in infant communicative action: Using dynamic systems theory to study individual utogenies. In J. Colombo & J. Fagan (Eds.), *Individual differences in infancy: Reliability, stability and prediction*. Hillsdale, NJ: Erlbaum.

Fogel, Alan (1991). *Infancy*. St. Paul, MN: West Publishing Company.

Gorski, P. (1985). Experience following premature birth. *Frontiers of Infant Psychiatry* (Vol. 2, pp. 145–151). New York: Basic Books.

Gorski, P. (1991). Developmental interventions during neonatal hospitalization. *Pediatric Clinics of North America, 38*, 1469–1479.

Graven, S. N., Bowen, Jr., F. W., Brooter, D., Eaton, A., Gravan, M. N., Hack, M., Hall, L. A., Hansen, N., Hurt, H., Kavalhvna, R., Little, G. A., Mahan, C., Morrow, G., III, Oehler, J. M., Poland, R., Ram, B., Sauve, R., Tayler, P. M., Ward, S. E., & Sommers, J. G. (1992). The high-risk infant environment: Part 1. The role of the neonatal intensive care unit in the outcome of high-risk infants. *Journal of Perinatalogy, 12*(2), 164–172.

High, D. C., & Gorski, P. (1985). Recording environmental influences on infant development in the intensive care nursery. In A. W. Gottfried & J. L. Gaiter (Eds.), *Infant stress under intensive care* (pp. 131–156). Baltimore: University Park Press.

Hiniker, P. K., & Moreno, L. A. (1994). *Developmentally supportive care: Theory and application.* Weymouth, MA: Childrens' Medical Ventures.

Johnston, C. C., & Stevens, B. (1990). Pain assessment in newborns. *Journal of Perinatal Neonatal Nursing, 4*(1), 41–52.

Korner, A. F., & Thom, V. A. (1990). *Neurobehavioral assessment of the preterm infant.* New York: The Psychological Corporation.

Lawson, J. R. (1988). Standards of practice and the pain of premature infants. *Zero to Three, 9*(2), 1–14.

Lefrak-Okikawa, L., & Lund, C. H. (1993). Nursing practice in the neonatal intensive care unit. In M. H. Klaus & A. A. Fanaroff (Eds.), *Care of the high-risk neonate* (pp. 212–227). Philadelphia: W. B. Saunders.

Levine, D., & Gordan, N. G. (1982). Pain in prelingual children and its evaluation by pain induced vocalization. *Pain, 14,* 85–93.

Lott, J. W. (1989). Developmental care of the preterm infant. *Neonatal Network, 7,* 21–28.

Mastropaolo, A. C., Consenstein, L., & Pergolizzi, J. J. (1994). One nursery: A scenario of change. In G. L. Ensher & D. A. Clark (Eds.), *Newborns at risk* (2nd ed. pp. 249–267). Gaithersburg, MD: Aspen.

Merenstein, G. B. (1994). Individualized developmental care: An emerging new standard for neonatal intensive care units? *Journal of the American Medical Association, 272,* 890–891.

Miller, M. Q., & Quinn-Hurst (1994). Neurobehavioral assessment of high risk infants in the neonatal intensive care unit. *The American Journal of Occupational Therapy, 48,* 506–513.

Rogers, M. C. (1992). Do the right thing. *New England Journal of Medicine, 326*(1), 55–56.

Tribotti, S. J., & Stein, M. (1992). From research to clinical practice: Implementing the NIDCAP. *Neonatal Network, 11,* 35–40.

Tronick, E., Scalon, K. B., & Scalon, J. W. (1987). Behavioral organization of the newborn preterm infant: Apathetic organization may not be normal. In *Infant stimulation: For whom, what kind, when and how much. Pediatric roundtable No.3.* Skillman, NJ: Johnson & Johnson.

VandenBerg, K. A. (1985). Revising the traditional model: An individualized approach to developmental interventions in the intensive care nursery. *Neonatal Network, 3,* 32–38.

Wells, P. W., DeBoard-Burns, M. B., Cook, R. C., & Mitchell, J. (1994). Growing up in the hospital: Part I, Let's focus on the child. *Journal of Pediatric Nursing, 9,* 66–73.

Williamson, P. S., & Williamson, M. C. (1983). Physiologic stress reduction by a local anesthetic during newborn circumcision. *Pediatrics, 71,* 36–40.

Wyly, M. V., & Allen, J. (1990). *Stress and coping in the intensive care unit.* Tuscon, AZ: Therapy Skill Builders.

Yecco, G. J. (1993). Neurobehavioral development and developmental support of premature infants. *Journal of Perinatal and Neonatal Nursing, 7,* 56–65.

■ CHAPTER 5
Hospital-Based Interventions for Premature Infants

*A touch is enough to let us know we're not
alone in the universe, even in sleep.*
Adrienne Rich

■ INTRODUCTION

Over the past two decades, a variety of behavioral interventions have been used with premature infants to compensate for their immaturity and their abbreviated interuterine experience. Some of these interventions provided extra sensory experiences, others attempted to modify the NICU environment or reduce stimulation to enhance preterm infant development.

The rationale behind these interventions has been guided by two schools of thought. The first school of thought argues that because premature infants are born too soon they are missing essential intrauterine experiences necessary for growth and development. Thus, it is necessary to simulate the peaceful aspects of the womb. Proponents of the other school of thought emphasize the differences between preterm and full-term infants. According to this group supplemental sensory stimulation is needed for catch-up of immature preterm infants with full-term infants.

Regardless of the intervention approach, the overriding concern is that premature low birthweight infants are at risk for subsequent behavioral and biological problems. By providing interventions in the NICU, it is hoped to ameliorate short- and long-term deleterious outcomes.

What concerns about preterm infant differences and outcomes have been identified in the research literature? Premature infants differ from full-term infants in a number of ways. Compared to healthy full-term infants, preterm infants exhibit different behavioral cues and are perceived as less competent by parents and NICU staff. Premature infants have less well-organized alert and sleep states, are more fussy, and have immature feeding patterns (Crnic, Rogozin, Greenberg, Robinson, & Basham 1983; Escalona, 1982). Very low birthweight infants often show massive behavioral and physiologic disorganization as well as inability to self-regulate due to their immature nervous system.

Although preterm infants' mortality rate has decreased, their survival is jeopardized by a myriad of medical problems (Als, 1992). There is continuing evidence that premature infants are at increased risk for a variety of biological and behavioral disorders. Recent estimates show that approximately 50% of infants discharged from neonatal intensive care units manifest minor neurodevelopmental disabilities such as attention disorders and learning and perceptual problems (McCormick, 1989). For very low birthweight infants (VBLW, i.e., less than 1500g) there are increased concerns about long-term developmental outcomes. Longitudinal studies show that major neurodevelopmental disorders such as mental retardation, sensory impairment, and cerebral palsy appear in 10 to 15% of this population (Bennett, 1990; Kopp, 1983).

Biological risk factors commonly seen in infants in the NICU, such as intraventricular hemorrhage (IVH) and bronchopulmonary dysplasia (BPD), are associated with poorer language skills, visual-perceptual motor problems, and learning difficulties (Klein, Hack, Gallagher, & Fanaroff, 1985; Vohr, 1991). Preterm infant outcome studies have provided evidence that in the preschool and elementary school years, a significant number of premature survivors are more prone to behavioral difficulties such as impulsiveness and disorganized social interactions (Escalona, 1984; Field, Dempsey, & Shuman, 1983; Goldberg, Corter, Lojkasek, & Minde, 1990).

Because of the multiplicity of risk factors that impinge on premature and low birthweight infants, environmental factors that may influence their developmental outcomes are being examined. Over the past 30 years, there have been many studies of the specific effects of supplemental tactile, auditory, visual, and kinesthetic stimulation during hospitalization on preterm growth and development. Skin-to-skin contact between infant and mother is currently being evaluated in terms of its affect on respiration, feeding, and digestive behaviors. Other investigators are studying the effects of minimal stimulation and therapeutic interventions prior and during medical interventions. In this chapter we will review the research on intervention strategies used with premature infants in the NICU. Current interventions strategies that are being used for developmental care will be described. Implications for clinical practice and family-focused initiatives will be highlighted.

■ BACKGROUND

The treatment model for premature infants in the neonatal intensive care nursery has been extended from a strictly medical focus to include early developmental interventions. These interventions focus on techniques that enhance preterm infants' behaviors, development, and coping abilities in the hospital and beyond. More and more has been learned about the effects of the NICU environment, invasive medical procedures, the immature neurology of preterm infants, and separation of infants and their families. As a result, health care professionals are now more aware of the need for using intervention strategies that will promote the preterm infants' quality of survival. These intervention techniques are termed "developmentally supportive care," which is care designed to recognize the individual needs of these infants and provide developmental support to enhance their well-being. The field of developmentally supportive care is rapidly growing and is derived from research begun in the 1960s on supplemental stimulation for preterms.

Since the 1960s, significant research on intervention has been conducted with the goal of optimizing the quality of care in the NICU, while at the same time ameliorating possible long-term developmental deficits. This focus of intervention in the NICU has changed significantly over the past 30 years, reflecting new knowledge and philosophical approaches to neonatal care.

In the 1960s and 1970s, the philosophy of neonatal developmental intervention studies was that premature infants needed supplemental stimulation (Hayes & Ensher, 1994). Increased sensory experiences were provided for premature infants who were thought to be sensorially deprived (Kramer, Chamorro, Green, & Knudtson, 1975; Solkoff & Matuszak, 1975). Sensory deprivation was believed to be the result of the lack of in utero stimulation as well as the isolation preterm infants supposedly experienced in the incubator (Blanchard, 1991; Scarr-Salpatek & Williams, 1973). Thus, investigators looked at ways that additional stimulation could compensate for preterm sensory deprivation.

Most of the studies published in this period described the outcomes of providing supplemental sensory stimulation such as tactile, visual, auditory, kinesthetic, and multimodal stimulation (Thurman, 1993). The methodology of these studies varied markedly. The sensory interventions used also varied considerably with regard to sequence, intensity, and duration of the stimulation. Sample selection and characteristics also varied. Infants used as subjects in the studies had a wide range of neurological maturity and gestational ages, but most excluded high-risk infants of very low birthweight (Ross,

1984). A wide variety of outcome measures were used including weight gain, length of hospitalization, performance on cognitive/sensory tasks after hospitalization, muscle tone, and degree of irritability and alertness (Bennett, 1987). Not surprisingly, the variability in the methodology of the research resulted in contradictory results and hampered the generalizing of the findings.

In 1976, Cornell and Gottfried challenged the sensory deprivation model. They argued that the supplemental stimulation research needed closer scrutiny since the actual level of stimulation received by preterm infants in the NICU had not yet been determined. They further argued that systematic observations and assessments of the extrauterine environment needed to be made prior to offering supplemental stimulation.

Yet, most of the preterm infant-focused stimulation studies published in the 1960s and 1970s reported at least one or more positive effects such as shorter hospital stay, decreased apnea spells, and weight gain. As Bennett (1990) pointed out in his review of this research "anything works." Surprisingly, there were few systematic replications of the systematic intervention protocols that had demonstrated positive outcomes for preterm infants. Thurman (1993) argued that most of the studies reported short-term outcomes and used healthy premature infants weighing 1000 grams or more, making it difficult to extrapolate the findings to sicker infant populations.

In the 1980s, research focused on the immediate and long-term impact of the technological care on premature babies. Rather than a source of sensory deprivation, the NICU was now viewed as an intrusive, overstimulating environment. Investigators looked at the effects of reducing excessive environmental stimulation in the NiCU (Gottfried & Gaiter, 1985).

There was also a growing awareness that both the quantity as well as the quality of sensory stimulation needed to be considered when initiating caregiving or medical interventions. The types of handling that accompanied medical and caregiving procedures was found to affect the physiological stability of fragile infants (Gorski, Hole, Leonard, & Martin, 1983). Hypoxemia was found to result from excessive handling due to interventions such as chest physical therapy, taking vital signs, suctioning, diaper change, feeding, and positioning (Long, Phillips, & Lucey, 1980). Hypoxemia occurs when there is inadequate oxygen in the blood, which can lead to hypoxia (insufficient oxygen to the tissues). Other investigators also noted decreases in preterm infants' blood oxygen levels in response to medical handling procedures (Murdoch & Darlow, 1984; Norris, Cambell, & Brenkert, 1982).

The impact of the effects of tactile stimulation was systematically studied by Blanchard, Pedneault, and Doray (1991). They found that in a sample of healthy preterm infants tactile stimulation did not result in hypoxemic episodes. In addition, oxygenation was improved in infants in the prone rather than supine position. In another study, the differential effects of heelsticks and tactile-kinesthetic message on blood oxygen levels was compared in stable preterm infants. Transcutaneous oxygen tension declined significantly more during heelstick procedures than during the message stimulation (Morrow et al., 1991). This suggests that medically stable premature infants may be able to tolerate handling, whereas forms of social touch may have adverse effects on sick preterm infants.

Handling or touching preterm infants was generally found to accompany medical and caregiving procedures rather than soothing them or providing touch contingent with their cues. Researchers began testing developmental interventions that minimized unnecessary handling and infant contacts. Still others examined the effects of sensory stimulation contingent on the behaviors of the infants (Barnard & Bee, 1983).

Als' pioneering work drew attention to the need to individualize interventions based on the behaviors of premature infants. Through careful assessment of individual infants self-regulating activities and stress cues, NICU caregivers can plan appropriate behavioral and environmental care (Als, Lester, Tronick, & Brazelton, 1982). Als and her colleagues proposed a conceptual model of synactive development in which interdependent subsystems gradually unfold and influence each other to form the behavioral organization of the preterm infant. These subsystems include the *autonomic system* that regulates visceral, respiration and color responses, *motor system* with its elements of posture, tone and movement, the *state system* which included the range of states of consciousness and their transitions, and the *interactional-attention system* which determines the capacity for degrees of alertness.

According to the synactive model, the growth and development of infants is determined by complex interplay between these subsystems and the environment. Within each subsystem, infants display stress signals and self-regulatory behaviors in response to environmental stimuli. Consequently, before sensory stimulation is reduced or added, the infant's competencies, stress levels, ability for self-regulation, and level of maturity must be assessed.

Several studies have documented the effectiveness of developmental care that support preterm infants' neurobehavioral organization. When NICU caregivers structured the neonatal care environment and modified their care of premature infants, significant outcome improvements were seen. These included shorter hospital stays, earlier nipple feeding, and fewer days on the ventilator. In addition, infants showed improved developmental status at discharge and at later follow-up evaluations (Als et al., 1994; Becker, Grunwald, Moorman, & Stuhr, 1991).

Als (1986) also proposed that developmental care in the NICU be designed to support individual infants and their parents. Other researchers investigated the effects of involving parents early on in aspects of caring for their infant in the NICU. Some intervention studies examined the effects of assisting parents to recognize and respond appropriately to their infant's communication signals, for example, alertness to the environment, stress signs, and social interaction cues. Mounting evidence supported the view that promoting parent visitation and positive parent-infant interactions are critical in enhancing the parent-infant relationship in the NICU (Brown et al., 1980).

Currently, more systematic methodology is being used to study the environmental-interactional networks of infants and their families in the neonatal intensive care unit (Miller & Hurst, 1994). Multisite, comprehensive investigations are examining the subtle effects of developmental interventions both in the NICU and after discharge on premature low birthweight infants and their families (Als, Lawhon, Duffy, McAnulty, Gibes-Grossman, & Blickman 1994; Heriza & Sweeney, 1990; Lefrak-Okikawa & Lund, 1993; Resnick, Armstrong, & Carter, 1988). The overall goal is to develop innovative intervention models that improve the outcomes of premature low birthweight infants (Jorgensen, 1993).

■ TACTILE AND KINESTHETIC STIMULATION

Since the 1960s investigators studied the effects of providing extra tactile and kinesthetic stimulation to premature infants. The rationale underlying these interventions was to improve premature infants' developmental and physiological well-being, for example, weight gain, increased head size, regulation of breathing or heart rate, alertness, and responsivity. The studies differed in methodology and measured outcomes, yet most of them demonstrated improved physiological or behavioral outcomes.

The supplemental stimulation model which guided the tactile/kinesthetic research in the 1960s was based on the research of Denenberg (1964) and Levine (1962). Through a systematic series of studies with rat pups, they found that the early experience of handling rat pups for 3 minutes daily modified adrenocortical function and reduced the rat pups' stress response to unfamiliar stimuli. Their animal model of early neonatal stimulation was applied in the preterm nursery in an attempt to understand the long- and short-term effects of supplemental stimulation on premature infants.

Hasselmeyer (1964) found that premature infants who were given extra tactile/kinesthetic stimulation such as stroking, cuddling, and rocking before and halfway between feedings were more quiescent than control infants who cried more. Solkoff, Jaffee, Weintraub, and Blase (1969) measured the effects of stroking preterm infants twice daily for 10-minute periods. Handled infants regained their birthweight more rapidly and showed improved motor development. Neal (1968) used rocking hammocks to provide continuous movement for low birthweight infants with the idea that the movement simulated that experienced by infants in utero. When tested at 36 weeks chronological age, the infants showed significantly increased weight gain compared to the control group. The experimental group also demonstrated higher visual and auditory response scores on the Graham-Rosenblith Neonatal Assessment. There was no difference in crying or irritability between the two groups.

Powell (1974) studied the effects of increased handling of low birthweight infants while hospitalized and following discharge. Subjects were handled for a 20-minute period twice a day beginning 72 hours after birth until they had regained their birthweight. They were then handled by the mother once a day for a 20-minute period. The type of handling used varied from touching to prolonged holding, depending on the infant. Control infants were given standard nursery care. Handled infants scored higher than the control group at 4 and 6 months on the Bayley Scales of Infant Development. The experimental group also regained their birthweight faster than the control infants, however there were no differences in height or weight gain in the follow-up at 2, 4 or 6 months. It was expected that encouraging mothers to hold their low birthweight infants would result in long-lasting differences in maternal behavior, yet there were no measurable differences found between mothers who were encouraged to touch their infants and those who were not. Powell did find that though maternal behaviors were unchanged, the mothers' perceptions of their infants were more positive. She concluded that hospitals were not doing enough to encourage parents to visit and handle their infants. Since the publication of this article in 1974, staff in neonatal intensive care units have made significant efforts to involve parents in infants' care.

Solkoff and Matuszak (1975) looked at the effects of stroking and flexing the arms and legs of five premature infants with birthweights less than 2000 grams. Compared to a control group, the stimulated infants demonstrated more positive ratings on the Brazelton Neonatal Assessment Scale. They were more alert, had better head control, better hand-to-mouth maneuvers, and were more easily comforted.

White and LaBarba (1976) provided extra tactile and kinesthetic stimulation to six premature, low birthweight infants. The stimulation was beyond that received by the control group who received standard nursing care. The stimulation involved rubbing the infant's neck, arms, legs, chest, shoulders, and back and flexing the arms and legs. Stimulation was administered every 15 minutes during a 4-hour period over 2 weeks. The experimental infants had increased formula intake during the treatment period and were eating more at the conclusion of treatment compared to controls. Experimental infants also had a more rapid weight gain over the treatment period. Similar findings were reported by Gausch (1981) who tested the effects of compensatory tactile and kinesthetic stimulation administered once daily on low birthweight infants. Treated infants had increased feeding intake and weight gain during the last 5 days of the 10 day treatment.

Kramer and associates (Kramer, Chamorro, Green, & Knudtson, 1975) studied the effects of extra tactile stimulation in the form of nonrhythmic stroking for 48 minutes daily on eight premature infants (mean gestational age 33 weeks). No significant differences were found between control and experimental infants on weight gain or rate of physical development. There was, however, a significant difference in the rate of social development of the control infants measured by the Bayley Scales of Infant Development.

Premature infants' cardiac and behavioral responses to a tactile stimulus during a sleep cycle were evaluated in a 1980 study (Rose, Schmidt, Riese, & Bridger, 1980). Three groups of infants were tested: 30 full-term infants, 30 nonintervened preterm infants and 30 intervened preterm infants. The tactile intervention consisted of daily massage of the shoulders, back, arms, hands, and feet of the infants administered within the first 2 weeks of life. The experimental preterm group showed increased cardiac responsiveness to the stimulation. The cardiac response was similar to that of full-term infants, although there were differences in duration of the cardiac acceleration between the full-term/preterm groups. The authors note that the intervention seemed to narrow the observed gap in behavioral responsivity between preterm and full-term infants.

The inconsistent findings of the tactile/kinesthetic stimulation on growth and development of stimulated preterm infants was pointed out in Field's (1986) review of supplemental stimulation studies with premature infants. Although some studies reported no differences in weight gain between the treatment and control infant groups, other studies showed that extra stimulation enhanced weight gain. Inconsistent findings were also found on the effects of tactile/kinesthetic stimulation on activity level and sleep/awake states. Field suggests that a number of variables might account for these differences across studies such as the weight and gestational age of the neonates, duration of hospital stay, and postnatal complications. The type of stimulation varied as well; in some studies hand stroking of the infants was used, whereas others employed finger stroking. Field noted that finger stroking, rather than soothing high-risk infants, could in fact be stressful, thus accounting for the differences reported in stroking studies.

Field and her colleagues conducted several studies to investigate the relationship of supplemental tactile/kinesthetic stimulation on growth and activity level of less mature, smaller and sicker premature infants. They used a random stratified sampling procedure to ensure comparability of the treatment and control groups with regards to gestational age, birthweight, and clinical complications. The tactile/kinesthetic stimulation included body stroking and passive movement of the limbs for three 15-minute periods a day for 10 days. Following treatment, the infant's behavioral states and activity level were observed and their neonatal behaviors were assessed using the Neonatal Behavioral Assessment Scale. The stimulated infants were more active and alert during the sleep/wake observations. They also averaged a 47% greater weight gain per day during treatment. The treated neonates showed more mature habituation, motor skills, and range of state behaviors as measured by the Brazelton scale (NBAS). Their hospital stay was 6 days shorter, suggesting that tactile/kinesthetic stimulation may be a cost effective way to reduce preterm infants' hospitalization (Field et al., 1986; Scafidi et al., 1986). Similar findings were reported in a follow-up study with 40 premature infants with a mean birthweight of 1176 grams.

The effects of providing tactile/kinesthetic stimulation similar to that normally provided by mothers was examined by Kilgo, Holder-Brown, Johnson, and Cook (1988). Stimulation was provided to a preterm treatment group for three 15-minute periods per day for 10 days. The weight gains and the performance of the treatment group on the NBAS increased significantly compared to the control group. There was no significant difference in the length of the hospital stay.

Message therapy was used by Field and colleagues with premature infants. Stable premature infants were randomly assigned to a message therapy group or control group. Following 10 days of three daily 15-minute massages, the massaged preterm infants gained significantly more weight. Infants who had experienced more complications before the study benefitted most from the therapy (Scafidi, Field, & Schanberg, 1993).

The effects of tactile/kinesthetic stimulation on sympathetic and adrenocortical function in preterm infants was investigated in a 1991 study. Preterm infants received tactile stimulation in the form of stroking for three 15-minute periods for 10 days and kinesthetic stimulation which consisted of five 1-minute segments of six passive flexion-extension motions. This stimulation was found to enhance maturation of the sympathetic nervous system and to facilitate weight gain and development in preterm infants (Kuhn et al., 1991).

Generally, the studies of the effects of tactile/kinesthetic stimulation demonstrate positive effects on weight gain of preterm infants. This type of stimulation also seems to enhance the organization of infants' state behaviors. The efficacy of tactile/kinesthetic stimulation results in improved performance on the Neonatal Behavioral Assessment Scale. The underlying mechanisms that facilitate these effects are still not well understood. Studies are needed that match the type, quantity, and length of the stimulation with varying levels of prematurity. The long-term benefits of tactile/kinesthetic stimulation must also be compared to the short-term benefits reported in most investigations.

■ VESTIBULAR STIMULATION

Beginning in the mid 1960s, investigations tested the idea that premature infants would benefit from additional vestibular stimulation. The assumption underlying this research was that preterm babies are deprived of the continuous rhythmic movement provided in the womb.

In one of the first vestibular stimulation experiments, Neal (1968) used a motorized hammock to rock an experimental infant group (28 to 32 weeks gestational age). When tested on the Graham-Rosenblith Scales at 36 weeks, the experimental infants scored higher on general maturation and motor development than the controls. Auditory and visual responsivity was augmented along with a significantly higher weight gain in the experimental group. In a second study, Neal (1977) rocked preterm infants in a motorized hammock then tested at 6 and 12 months of age on the Bayley Scales of Infant Development. By 12 months, all of the infants in the motorized hammock group scored above the 50th percentile on the test compared to only 80% of the control group.

The effects of increased vestibular stimulation on preterm infants was systematically examined by Korner and associates. They proposed that the use of water beds would provide stimulation that resembled intrauterine conditions. Oscillating water beds were used as the stimulus. The effects of the waterbeds on infants' respiratory patterns and other physiologic systems were then measured. In one study they placed infants on a waterbed for a total of 7 days, and they found no significant differences between the experimental and control groups in weight gain, incidence of vomiting, respiratory rate, or mean daily heart rate. There were, however, significantly fewer apnea episodes in the experimental group (Korner, Kremer, Haffner, & Cosper, 1975). A follow-up study on the effects of waterbed floatation on the respiration and sleep of eight apneic preterm infants showed that apnea was significantly reduced when the infants were on water beds (Korner, Guilleminault, Van den Hood, & Baldwin, 1978).

Korner, Schneider, and Forest (1983) examined the effects of vestibular-proprioceptive stimulation on the neurobehavioral development of 20 premature infants. The treatment group was less irritable, were better able to attend to visual and auditory stimuli, and were more often visually alert, promoting these investigators to conclude that vestibular-proprioceptive stimulation may enhance neuorbehavioral development of preterm infants.

Korner, Ruppel, and Rho (1982) assessed the sleep patterns and mobility of theophylline-treated preterm infants with BPD (26–32 weeks PGA) following four days on an oscillating waterbed and during the similar time on a standard mattress. The infants served as their own controls. The waterbed floatation increased the calm sleep states of the infants and decreased jittery movements of their extremities. Similarly, Pelletier, Short, and Nelson (1985) described significantly increased hand-to-mouth movements and decreased body arching and startles in preterm infants (29 to 33 weeks gestation) placed on oscillating waterbeds following gavage feedings. The infant control group was placed on standard mattresses.

Barnard (1973) combined vestibular stimulation in the form of oscillating beds with heartbeat recordings for a 15-minute period each hour during the 33rd and 34th weeks post gestational age. When tested at 35 weeks, the experimental group scored higher on the neurological maturation scale of the Dubowitz, Dubowitz, and Goldberg Clinical Assessment of Gestational Age. Infants in the experimental group spent more time in quiet sleep state than did the controls.

Other investigators documented the effects of vestibular stimulation on sleep/wake states in premature infants. Burns, Deddish, Burns, and Hatcher (1983) used oscillating waterbeds and taped recordings of interuterine sounds. The experimental group of preterm infants scored significantly better in motor and state organization. The experimental group also had a significant drop in active sleep. Edelman, Kraemer, and Korner (1982) found vestibular stimulation decreased preterm infants' irritability as well as increased quiet sleep states.

Most of the research on vestibular stimulation employed oscillating beds or waterbeds. Overall positive outcomes have been reported. Vestibular stimulation has been shown to increase quiet sleep states in premature infants, increase weight gains, and decrease apnea and bradycardia episodes (Tuck, Monin, Duvivier, May, & Vert, 1982). Better motoric organization and neurologic development has been demonstrated in several studies. Aside from the vestibular input, some clinicians argue that the use of waterbeds is beneficial. Waterbeds may provide containment for infants, as well as alleviate the head-flattening common to preterm infants.

■ AUDITORY STIMULATION

There is little research on the effects of auditory stimulation on premature infants due to the difficulties of managing the experimental procedures with preterm infants. The following studies are examples of the research used in assessing this sensory intervention.

Katz (1971) used 5-minute tape recordings of mother's voice, six times daily at 2-hour intervals. This experimental procedure began on the fifth day of life and continued until the infants reached 36 weeks gestational age. At 36 weeks gestational age, infants in the experimental group had more optimal scores in general maturation and increased auditory and visual ability as measured by the Graham-Rosenblith Behavior Scale.

Segal (1972) played tape recordings of mother's voice using a speaker placed in the baby's incubator. The recording was played for a 30-minute period every day until the infants reached 36 weeks gestational age. At 36 weeks the experimental group (N = 30) and control group (N = 30) were presented a variety of auditory stimuli including the mother's voice, an unfamiliar female voice, and white noise. The infants' cardiac response to the stimuli was measured. The experimental group showed an accelerated heart rate to the white noise, indicating a neurological recognition of the unfamiliar. Across trials, the experimental group showed a decrease in heart response compared to an irregular response of the control group. This suggests an ability to habituate or adapt to a novel stimulus. It was also found that during a crying state, those infants exposed to mother's voice as part of the experimental procedure had a significantly decreased response to their mother's voice and unfamiliar female voice.

These findings indicate that premature infants have the capacity to attend to the human voice even when crying and show adaptive responses to different auditory stimuli when exposed to systematic auditory stimulation early in life. Although more research in this area is needed, these results support current clinical interventions that encourage parents to sit by the bedsides of very early neonates and speak softly to them.

∎ MULTIMODAL STIMULATION

Multimodal stimulation studies with preterm infants have employed two or more sensory modalities including visual, tactile, vestibular, auditory, and kinesthetic stimuli. The studies vary considerably in terms of design factors, sample size, and outcome measures. Beneficial effects have been demonstrated in all of the studies, some of which are highlighted below.

In one of the earliest multimodal stimulation studies, Scarr-Salapatek and Williams (1973) had nursery staff take low birthweight infants between 1300 grams and 1800 grams to a special intervention room for feedings where they talked to, rocked, stroked, patted, and looked at the infants. Visual stimulation in the form of mobiles was provided both within and outside of the incubator for those infants who could not be removed from the incubator. The goal was to provide stimulation that approximated optimal home stimulation. The stimulation intervention was introduced for eight 30-minute sessions daily. The stimulation program was continued weekly in the home for 1 year after discharge. The experimental group showed a significant weight gain compared to the control group while in the nursery. When tested on the Catell Infant Intelligence Scale at 1 year, the experimental group showed significantly higher scores.

Leib, Benfield, and Guidubaldi (1980) also attempted to simulate the multimodal sensory environment of the home. Infants in the experimental treatment group were rubbed or touched during gavage feedings. Later, during nipple feedings, nurses rocked them and sang or talked to them. Mobiles and music boxes were placed in or near the cribs. At a 6-month developmental follow-up, the experimental infants showed an increase in scores on the Bayley Scales of Infant Development.

Kramer and Pierpont (1976) found that preterm infants placed on water beds and then rocked rhythmically to auditory stimuli showed accelerated head growth, nippled earlier, and were more active than the control infants. More recently, Barnard and Bee (1983) used vestibular stimulation (oscillating bed) accompanied by taped heartbeat recording to resemble the intrauterine environment. The intervention was provided in three treatment modes: fixed interval stimulation given 15 minutes each hour, self-activating stimulation given after every 90 seconds of inactivity and quasi-self-activating stimulation given for 15 minutes after 90 seconds of inactivity limited to one stimulation per hour. Infants in the treatment groups had decreased rates of activity and fewer abnormal reflexes compared to the control group. When tested on the Bayley Scales of Infant Development at 24 months, treatment infants had better scores than the control infants.

Resnick, Armstrong, and Carter (1988) tested a program of hospital-based multimodal stimulation and home-based developmental interventions designed to promote optimal high-risk infant development and parent-infant communication. Infants in the treatment group weighed 1800 grams or more. The in-hospital intervention included an auditory tape of heartbeat, classical music, and parent's voice; total body massage; passive range of motion; exercise on a waterbed; rocking; and en face stimulation with face or objects and oral stimulation prior to feeding. Following discharge, twice monthly home-based stimulation activities were modeled and guided by a child development specialist. Follow-up evaluations at 6 and 12 months indicated that the infants in the treatment group scored higher on the Bayley Scales of Infant Development. There were significant positive effects on parent-infant interactions as measured by the Greenspan-Lieberman Observations System.

■ OTHER SENSORY STIMULATION

Nonnutritive Sucking

Sucking is a simple reflex that is present in healthy full-term newborns. The sucking reflex is essential to an infant's survival. The sucking action consists of a pattern of combining the use of positive and negative pressure. Newborns suck in bursts and then they pause. Gradually, neonatal sucking evolves into a more mature sucking response.

Newborn sucking patterns can elicit mutual turntaking between the infant and caregiver. Often during the pause the caregiver will jiggle the infant. Although the jiggle actually retards sucking, the infant resumes, thus continuing a turntaking interaction with the caregiver.

The sucking response has been observed as early as 17 weeks gestational age (Dubignon, Campbell, & Patington, 1969). By 28 weeks the sucking, rooting, and swallowing reflexes are established but not fully matured (Amiel-Tison, 1968). Coordination of sucking, swallowing, and breathing occurs at approximately 34 weeks gestational age. Healthy premature infants have the suck and swallow reflex by 32 to 34 weeks; however, younger premature infants lack this ability. Premature infants usually cannot use sucking to bottle feed until around 35 weeks (Brake, Fifer, Alfasi, & Fleischman, 1988). The opportunity for sucking, common to full-term newborns, is not always available for young premature infants who are tube fed. Beyond 34 weeks gestation, healthy premature infants can coordinate sucking with breathing and swallowing (Meier, 1993). Continuous and intermittent sucking phases are typical of stable, healthy preterm infants 34 weeks and beyond. These sucking patterns are similar to those of full-term infants (Glass & Wolf, 1994).

Providing nonnutritive sucking opportunities for preterm infants is being investigated as a safe, cost effective means to promote self-regulatory behavior, calm infants during intrusive medical interventions, and to facilitate later bottle feeding (Anderson, Burroughs, & Measel, 1983; Field et al., 1982). Nonnutritive sucking can be done by placing a pacifier in the infant's mouth.

Field et al. (1982) gave pacifiers to premature, low birthweight (less than 1800 grams) infants with respiratory problems during all tube feedings. The treatment group had higher average weight gain and shorter hospital stay than the control group. Further, the treatment group had fewer days of tube feedings than the control group and were easier to feed in later bottle feeds. A longitudinal follow-up of the infants in the nonnutritive group showed that they had greater weight and head circumferences than infants in the control group at 12 and 24 months. The authors suggest that nonnutritive sucking opportunities facilitates quieting and central nervous system organization.

The positive effects of nonnutritive sucking on premature infants has been documented in a number of studies. Nonnutritive sucking improves oxygenation of premature infants (Anderson et al., 1983). It promotes quiet sleep with less time in active sleep with fewer state transitions (Measel & Anderson, 1979; Woodson, Drinkwin, & Hamilton, 1985). Sucking reduces expenditure of energy in fussing and excessive movement, thus facilitating growth (Field, 1986). Nonnutritive sucking affects movement, state regulation, and arousal (Kimble & Dempsey, 1992; Pickler & Frankel, 1995). Provision of pacifiers during heelsticks reduces the physiological response caused by this stressful procedure (Field & Goldson, 1984). One of the more important outcomes of the simple intervention of nonnutritive sucking is rapid weight gain and earlier hospital discharge for preterm infants (Bernbaum, Pereira, Watkins, & Peckham, 1983; Field et al., 1982). Nonnutritive sucking has been shown to help infants soothe themselves. Kling (1989) points out that in NICUs nonnutritive sucking is being used to reduce discomfort and pain.

It has been suggested that the mechanism responsible for improved weight gain, more rapid transition from gavage to bottle feeding, and shorter hospitalization found with nonnutritive sucking is increased gastric secretion. This secretion stimulates acid secretion and growth of gastric mucosa (Pickler & Terrell, 1994).

Kangaroo Care

Another type of tactile stimulation currently being used in neonatal intensive care units is known as Kangaroo Care. **Kangaroo care** or skin-to-skin contact is a method of placing diaper clad infants in an upright position between their mother breasts or on one breast (Anderson, Marks, & Wahlberg, 1986). Kangaroo care was introduced by pediatricians Rey and Martinez in Bogota, Colombia in 1979 as an alternative to hospital care where incubators and warmers were scarce, infection was common, and infant mortality high (Whitelaw & Sleath, 1985). Mothers acted as "human incubators" for their preterm infants at home. This practice was reported to have positive outcomes for infants as small as 1000 grams living in impoverished homes, as well as facilitating parent-infant attachment.

Early reports of the effectiveness of this practice prompted a closer look at kangaroo care. Investigators visited Bogota to observe kangaroo care first hand. Research projects were implemented in the United States and Europe on aspects of skin-to skin care (Anderson,1991). Kangaroo care began to be implemented in conjunction with standard intensive care for preterm infants in NICUs in several Western European countries, particularly Scandinavia as well as the United States (Anderson, 1989; Laine, 1987).

With the adoption of kangaroo care came variations and refinements to the method. Complete kangaroo care is described as holding baby skin-to-skin with self-regulatory access to breast feeding. Fathers also may hold the baby kangaroo style. Four categories of kangaroo care currently in practice are described by Anderson (1991). **Late kangaroo care** begins after the baby has stabilized and is off the ventilator. This means it begins days or weeks after birth. **Early kangaroo care** begins with infants who are stabilized within a few hours or days after birth. **Immediate kangaroo care** is initiated after early intensive care, which is approximately 1 week following birth. Babies may still be on ventilators or have apnea episodes in this category. Very early kangaroo care begins during the first minutes after birth. Babies are returned to their mothers who place the baby between their breasts. The infants then stay near their mother, either in an incubator or in the same bed.

What is the evidence that kangaroo care is beneficial to preterm infants or their parents? A number of research studies as well as descriptive analyses of kangaroo care have been conducted (Anderson, 1991; Whitelaw, 1990). Generally, the conclusions from the research demonstrate that kangaroo care is an intervention that benefits both premature infants and their parents.

A randomized, control study of 71 mothers and preterm very low birthweight infants showed that skin contact for a mean of 36 minutes a day increased the duration of lactation in the skin-to-skin group. At 6 months of age these infants were reported to have significantly less crying than the control infants (Whitelaw, Heisterkamp,

Sleath, Acolet, & Richards, 1988). Laine (1987) reported similar findings of improved lactation with skin-to-skin contact of 20 to 60 minutes a day for 3 to 4 weeks. An additional finding was that the mothers also verbalized feelings of satisfaction with their baby. Premature infants who experienced skin-to-skin contact for three consecutive feeding days before hospital discharge had more quiet than active sleep (Ludington, 1990). Increased oxygenation and thermal regulation were found to be related to kangaroo care (Acolet, Sleath, & Whitelaw, 1989). In several studies of premature infants and mothers, kangaroo care has been shown to increase mothers' confidence in breast feeding and monitoring their infant. Kangaroo care also increases maternal self-esteem, sense of mastery and feelings of closeness to their infant (Affonso, Bosque, Wahlberg, & Brady, 1993; Affonso, Wahlberg, & Persson, 1989).

Investigations involving randomized clinical trials are currently in progress at sites throughout the United States. Long-term outcomes of kangaroo care as well as the physiologic effects of skin-to-skin care still need evaluation. The psychological outcomes for mother and father and possible ways to facilitate kangaroo care as a parent intervention in the NICU warrant closer research scrutiny.

Conclusion

What can we conclude from the sensory stimulation research? Does supplemental stimulation of infants in the NICU make a difference for the well-being of premature infants? Almost all of the studies reported beneficial effects for preterm infant development. Those studies, which measured the impact of the intervention on parents of premature infants, found that parents felt more satisfaction and self-confidence in caring for their infant. However, these results must be qualified because of the problems with the research designs, methodologies, subject selection, terms of duration of the intervention, dependent measures, and assumptions underlying the research.

Studies that examined the effects of one sensory modality for example, auditory vestibular stimulation, varied markedly in terms of the stimulus used. For example, vestibular stimulation in some studies was a waterbed, but in others a motorized rocking bed or a nurse or parent rocked the infant. The intervention studies that reported positive effects of more than one sensory interventions also used different types, amounts, and combination of stimulus interventions, which makes it difficult to assess the effectiveness of these interventions (Gilkerson, Gorski, & Panitz, 1990).

The sample populations used in these studies also varied considerably. Most of the research was done with relatively healthy preterm infants. Usually very low birthweight or infants with severe problems were excluded as subjects. Infants of scattered gestational ages were used in some studies, while in other studies the infants studied were of one narrow gestational age. Individual infants' responsivity to environmental stimuli is not considered in this research despite the fact that infants of the same gestational age demonstrate different levels of toleration to extraneous stimulation.

Comparing studies using supplemental stimulation is further hampered by the problem of the differences in the onset, duration, and frequency of the intervention. In some cases sensory stimulation was begun several days after birth, whereas others began the intervention sometime after the infants were stabilized (Masi, 1979). Some of the interventions were of short duration, for example, several days, and some continued through discharge and transition to home. The application of the intervention differed widely from making it contingent on the infant's response or on a daily or hourly schedule or prior to feeding.

A variety of outcome measures (dependent variables) have been reported in this research (Bennett, 1990; Heriza & Sweeney, 1990). Some investigators document developmental or behavioral changes such as auditory responsivity, state regulation, activity level, or muscle tone. Other studies employ medical outcome measures such as weight gain, oxygenation, frequency of apnea and bradycardia episodes, head growth, or length of hospitalization. Still other studies use parental outcome measures to assess the intervention's effectiveness. These measures often monitor parent visitation, parent satisfaction, and parent infant interaction. The inconsistency of the outcome measures used make it difficult to accurately link them to specific interventions. Although positive benefits of sensory stimulation are reported in this literature, clinicians should remain sensitive to the methodological weaknesses of this research before introducing supplemental stimulation into medical protocols.

The impetus for researchers in the 1990s is for more systematic studies of the effects of developmental intervention programs on infants and their families. Answers are being sought to such questions as: What specific stimulation has positive benefits? What are the long- and short-term outcomes of added stimulation? Does stimulation provided by parents facilitate the parent-infant relationship? The new approach of integrating individualized developmental care after assessing each infants' capabilities holds promise (Als, 1986). Further, the advent of the family-centered model in NICUs should provide opportunities to investigate the efficacy of family focused, developmental care.

■ CLINICAL APPLICATIONS

Currently, neonatal intervention programs are being designed to address specific individual needs of fragile preterm infants (Creger, 1989). Rather than apply sensory stimulation indiscriminently, NICU health providers structure individualized care plans. Some guidelines for developing individual care interventions are described in this section.

When structuring an appropriate intervention for preterm infants, the first step is to correctly read infant stress and self-regulation signs. This requires knowing what to look for in the infant's appearance and behaviors. The second step is to determine whether an environmental change or direct infant intervention should be implemented. In some cases, the caregiver should simply allow the infants to gain control through the use of their self-regulatory behaviors. The third step is to structure careful environmental changes to minimize infant stress and encourage self-regulatory behaviors. Alternatively, a behavioral-developmental intervention may be introduced—one that focuses on assisting infants to reduce their stress or one that promotes attachment in more intact infants. These procedures involve developmental management of the infant and require that the caregivers know the infant well and know how to assess autonomic and physiologic stress signs.

Implementing Individualized Developmental Interventions in the NICU

Developmental interventions for high-risk infants in neonatal intensive care units must be applied with caution. The key is to individualize—to tailor approaches to each infant, building on a baseline knowledge of that infant's capabilities. Health professionals should first observe, then assess, the infant's physiologic and behavioral signs of compromise; that is, what stresses an infant and what, if any, coping mechanisms are available and used. The infant's medical condition and vulnerability also must be considered. Often the high-risk infant is neurologically and behaviorally disorganized and thus unable to cope with the stress of any environmental stimulation.

For some infants, any stimulation or intervention is inappropriate. Even necessary medical procedures may tax these infants' already overtaxed systems, resulting in stress overload. Infants become aroused during medical procedures, may become disorganized, and may show signs of behavioral disorganization for as long as 5 minutes after the procedure is over (Gorski, Hole, Hole, & Martin, 1983).

In many NICUs, minimal stimulation signs are placed near the incubators of very sick premature infants to alert medical staff of the need to provide a less stressful environment for the infant. Minimal stimulation includes eliminating or reducing handling or touching the infant, carefully planning medical interventions to match the infant's state, and providing the infant with a quiet environment.

What caregivers consider a nonstressful intervention may in fact be stressful for the infant. Some infants "fall apart," for example, show stress signs and physiologic instability, during or after a medical intervention. The infant's physiological, motor, and autonomic systems must be stable before any stimulation is applied. The timing and content of the interventions are crucial in terms of their positive or negative effects on an infant's well-being. The strategies selected should calm the fussy infant, facilitate parent involvement with their infants, or assist infants in self-regulation (Als et al., 1986).

Before planning and implementing interventions in the NICU, several questions should be asked:

1. *How well do I know the infant?* Infants are individual. They have their own ways of responding, alerting to the environment, using stimulation, becoming stressed, and recovering from stress. Some infants are more irritable than others, have more robust states, show better motor tone, or are more active. Some infants will become quickly disorganized, while others are able to tolerate more in the environment. Others are unable to tolerate any stimulation at all, and the intervention should be *no* intervention! The more time spent watching and assessing individual differences in infants will result in more appropriate interventions. If the answer to the question of "How well do I know the infant?" is "Not very well," then more time should be spent carefully assessing the infant's capabilities.

2. *What is the infant's gestational age and medical condition?* If the infant is very young and fragile, *any* stimulation probably is excessive. As the infant matures, there are increased capabilities and a greater ability to manage environmental stimulation. The infant's gestational age, medical condition, and individual responses should be used as guideposts for intervention.

3. *What are the signs of infant state?* While infant behavioral states are usually easy to identify in a full-term baby, often it is difficult to distinguish states in the preterm infant. For the very young preterm infant, only two states, deep sleep and active sleep, are present. Often the physiological and

behavioral signs of the infant state are subtle and transient. Recognizing them in a preterm infant takes practice. Identification of infant state is crucial in determining the appropriateness of the intervention. For example, if the infant signs indicate a deep sleep state, introducing an intervention should be discouraged.

4. *Is the infant able to self-regulate the states?* A healthy term neonate regularly moves from state to state and is capable of regulating states to match environmental stimulation. Even within normal infant populations, there are variations in state regulation. In premature infants, however, the ability to regulate states may be absent or minimal. In the very young preterm infant, there is not much evidence of state regulation across the various behavioral states. Premature infants older than 34 weeks begin to show some state regulation and movement across the six behavioral states, but this may depend on the infant's condition and medical status. The ability to regulate states and move from state to state becomes more pronounced with older, healthier infants. Once some degree of state regulation is observed in infants, it is possible to provide either arousal or soothing techniques to assist the preterm infant to regulate states.

5. *Are infant states clear or disorganized?* The clarity and robustness of state behaviors are clues to an infant's ability to cope. An organized state in which behaviors are identifiable and sustained is an indicator that the infant's autonomic nervous system is capable of regulation. As states become more organized, caregivers can better match their behaviors to that of infants. Infants in turn are able to shut out stimulation or maintain social interaction. For example, an infant who is capable of sustaining alertness to the caregiver's face is far more capable of social interactions that an infant who becomes hyperaroused after several seconds of looking at the caregiver.

6. *Does the infant transition across states smoothly?* Transitions from state to state involve a complex interaction of the infant's central nervous system and autonomic nervous system. The somatic changes that result sensitize the infant to any stimulation. Interventions that assist infants to move from one state to another must include monitoring infant responses. Stop interventions if signs of stress overload appear. Often these stress signs can be so subtle that they can be missed. Color changes, movements, or physiologic indicators such as irregular respiration show that the infant has

had "too much." Accurately reading subtle stress signs may well prevent the occurrence of more obvious signs of stress such as apnea or bradycardia.

7. *What is the capacity of the individual infant to handle stimulation and recover from overload?* Each intervention must match the capacity and individuality of each infant. Infants who are more intact are better able to cope with external and internal demands. Other infants may become easily overloaded and show signs that they are stressed and out of control. It is important to remember that infants may not always be consistent in their ability to respond to environmental stimulation. For example, an infant may be judged as a reliable responder, yet be unable to adequately recover when a caregiving intervention closely follows a medical intervention.

8. *What are the infant's readiness signals to interact with the caregiver?* The NICU health professional must know and be able to read each infant's interaction cues, and the strength of these cues must be accurately measured. The cues may be body positioning, movement, cooing, looking at the caregiver's face, or sustaining an attentional gaze. Some fragile infants do give interaction cues to their caregivers, but they are brief and weak. Sometimes the signals are not for interaction but rather to say "Please leave me alone." Weak signals probably mean that the infant does not have the capacity to sustain an interaction and cannot tolerate an intervention. Stronger, more defined signals may allow a caregiver to provide a multisensory intervention that lasts a longer time.

■ SUMMARY

For the past 30 years, sensory stimulation of the preterm infant has been investigated. The assumption guiding the early research was that the preterm infants were in a state of sensory deprivation because of being born too soon. Supplemental stimulation was needed to offset the sensory deprivation experienced in the extrauterine environment.

During the 1960s and 1970s supplemental stimulation programs for premature infants were studied using a single or multimodal sensory modality. Despite the variability in the studies and the methodological problems of the research, most studies demonstrated beneficial effects.

Investigators began to question the validity of the sensory deprivation model. In the 1980s research focused on the quality of the infant's sensory experience. More careful attention was given to the effects of the NICU environment and caregiving experiences of the infant. Infants in the intensive care nursery were thought to experience overstimulation rather than deprivation.

Clinicians in the 1990s began investigations of the outcomes of individualized care. Sensory interventions were adapted to each infant's specific medical status, level of maturation, and self-regulatory capabilities. The direct involvement of parents in facilitating their infant's optimal development has also been a focus of current research.

Attention is now being given to selecting intervention strategies appropriate for each infant in the NICU. Infant states, level of arousal, gestational age, and medical conditions are considered in order to match interventions with the infant's physiologic and behavioral levels. Caregivers must know the range of interventions appropriate for fragile infants and if or when to initiate intervention. Recognizing the family role in intervention and facilitating parent involvement is essential to infants' long-term well-being.

■ REFERENCES

Acolet, D., Sleath, K., & Whitelaw. (1989). Oxygenation, heart rate and temperature in very low birth weight infants during skin-to-skin contact with their mothers. *Actor Paediatricia Scandinavica, 78,* 189–193.

Affonso, D. D., Bosque, E., Walhberg, V., & Brady, J. P. (1993). Reconciliation and healing for mother through skin-to-skin contact provided in an American tertiary level intensive care nursery. *Neonatal Network, 12,* 25–32.

Affonso, D. D., Wahlberg, V., & Persson, B. (1989). Exploration of mother's reactions to the kangaroo method of prematurity care. *Neonatal Network, 7,* 43–51.

Als, H. (1986). Synactive model of neonatal behavioral organization: Framework for the assessment and support of the neurobehavioral development of the premature infant and his parents in the environment of 8th neonatal intensive care unit. In J. K. Sweeney (Ed.), *The high-risk neonate: Developmental therapy perspectives* (pp. 3–55). New York: The Haworth Press.

Als, H. (1992). Individualized, family-focused developmental care for the very low-birthweight preterm infant in the NICU. In S. L. Friedman & M. D. Sigman (Eds.), *The psychological development of low-birthweight children* (pp. 341–388). Norwood, NJ: Ablex Press.

Als, H., Lawhon, G., Brown, E., Gibes, R., Duffy, F. H., McAnulty, G. B. & Blickman, J. G. (1986). Individualized behavioral and environmental care for the very low birth weight preterm infant at high risk for broncho pulmonary dysplasia: Neonatal intensive care unit and developmental outcome. *Pediatrics, 78,* 1123–1132.

Als, H., Lawhon, G., Duffy, F., McAnulty, G., Gibes-Grossman, R., & Blickman, J. (1994). Individualized developmental care for the very low birthweight preterm infant. *Journal of the American Medical Association, 272,* 853–858.

Als, H., Lester, B. M., Tronick, E. C., & Brazelton, T. B. (1982). Toward a research instrument for the assessment of preterm infant behavior. In H. E. Fitzgerald, B. E. Lester, & M. W. Yogman (Eds.), *Theory and research in behavioral pediatrics Vol. 1* (pp 35–63) New York: Plenum Publishers.

Amiel-Tison, C. (1968). Neurological evaluation of the maturity of newborn infants. *Archives of Disease in Childhood, 43*, 89–93.

Anderson, G. C. (1989). Skin-to-skin Kangaroo care in Western Europe. *American Journal of Nursing, 89*, 662–666.

Anderson, G. C. (1991). Current knowledge about skin-to-skin (Kangaroo) care for preterm infants. *Journal of Perinatalogy, 11*, 216–226.

Anderson, G. C., Burroughs, S. K., & Measel, C. P. (1983). Non nutritive sucking opportunities: A safe and effective treatment for premature infants. In T. Field & A. Sostek (Eds.), *Infants born at risk: Physiological, perceptual and cognitive processes* (pp. 129–145). New York: Grune & Stratton.

Anderson, G. C., Marks, E. A., & Wahlberg, V. (1986). Kangaroo care for premature infants. *American Journal of Nursing, 86*, 807–809.

Barnard, K. (1973). The effect of stimulation on the sleep behavior of the premature infant. *Communicating Nursing Research, 6*, 12–40.

Barnard, K. E., & Bee, H. L. (1983). The impact of temporally patterned stimulation on the development of preterm infants. *Child Development, 54*, 1156–1167.

Becker, P. T., Grunwald, P. C., Moorman, J., & Stuhr, S. (1991). Outcome of developmentally supportive nursery care for very low birthweight infants. *Nursing Research, 40*, 150–155.

Bennett, F. C. (1987). The effectiveness of early intervention for infants at increased biological risk. In M. J. Guralnick & F. C. Bennett (Eds.), *The effectiveness of early intervention for at-risk and handicapped children* (pp. 79–112). Orlando, FL: Academic Press.

Bennett, F. C. (1990). Recent advances in developmental intervention for biologically vulnerable infants. *Infants and Young Children, 3*, 33–40.

Bernbaum, J. C., Periera, G. R., Watkins, J. B., & Peckham, G. C. (1983). Non nutritive sucking during gavage feedings enhances growth and maturation in premature infants. *Pediatrics, 71*, 41–45.

Blanchard, Y. (1991). Early intervention and stimulation of the hospitalized preterm infant. *Infants and Young Children, 4*, 76–84.

Blanchard, Y., Pedneault, M., & Doray, B. (1991). Effects of tactile stimulation on physical growth and hypoexemia in preterm infants. *Physical & Occupational Therapy in Pediatrics, 11*, 37–52.

Brake, S. C., Fifer, W. P., Alfasi, G., & Fleischman, A. (1988). The first nutritive sucking response of premature newborns. *Infant Behavior and Development, 11*, 1–19.

Brown, J., LaRossa, M., Aylward, G., Davis, D. J., Rutherford, P. K., & Bakeman, R. (1980). Nursery-based intervention with prematurely born babies and their mothers: Are there effects. *Journal of Pediatrics, 97*, 487–491.

Burns, K. A., Dessish, R. B., Burns, W. J., & Hatcher, R. P. (1983). Use of oscillating waterbeds and rhythmic sounds for premature infant stimulation. *Developmental Psychology, 19*, 746–751.

Cornell, E. H., & Gottfried, A. W. (1976). Intervention with premature human infants. *Child Development, 47,* 32–39.

Creger, P. J. (1989). *Developmental interventions for preterm and high-risk infants.* Tucson, AZ: Therapy Skill Builders.

Crnic, K. A., Rogozin, A. S., Greenberg, M. T., Robinson, N. M., & Basham, R. B. (1983). Social interaction and developmental competence of preterm and full-term infants during the first year of life. *Child Develoment, 54,* 119-121.

Denenberg, V. H. (1964). Critical periods, stimulus input, and emotional reactivity: A theory of infantile stimulation. *Psychological Review, 71,* 335–351.

Dubignon, J. M., Campbell, D., & Patington, M. W. (1969). The development of non nutritive sucking in premature infants. *Biology of the Neonate, 14,* 270–278.

Edelman, A. H., Kraemer, H. C., & Korner, A. F. (1982). Effects of compensatory movement stimulation on the sleep-wake bahaviors of preterm infants. *Journal of the American Academy of Child Psychiatry, 21,* 555–559.

Escalona, S. K. (1982). Babies at double hazard: Early development of infants at biologic and social risk. *Pediatrics, 70,* 670–676.

Escalona, S. K. (1984). Social and other environmental influences on the cognitive and personality development of low birthweight infants. *American Journal of Mental Deficiency, 88,* 508–512.

Field, T., Dempsey, J., & Shuman, H. H. (1983). Five year follow-up of preterm respiratory distress syndrome and post-term post maturity syndrome infants. In T. Field & A. Sostek (Eds.), *Infants born at risk: Physiological, perceptual and cognitive processes* (pp. 317–335). New York: Grune & Stratton.

Field, T., & Goldson, E. (1984). Pacifying effects of non nutritive sucking on term and preterm neonates during heelsticks. *Pediatrics, 74,* 1012–1015.

Field, T., Ignatoff, E., Stringer, J. B., Brenner, M., Greenberg, R., Windmayer, S., & Anderson, G. C. (1982). Non nutritive sucking during tube feedings. Effects on preterm neonates in an intensive care unit. *Pediatrics, 70,* 381–384.

Field, T. M. (1986). Interventions for premature infants. *Journal of Pediatrics, 109,* 183–191.

Field, T. M., Schanberg, S. M., Scafidi, F., Bauer, C. R., Vega-Lahr, N., Garcia, R., Nystrom, J., & Kuhn, C. M. (1986). Tactile kinesthetic stimulation effects on preterm neonates. *Pediatrics, 77,* 654–658.

Gausch, P. (1981). Effects of tactile and kinesthetic stimulation on premature infants. *Journal of Obstetric and Gyneologic Neonatal Nursing, 10,* 34–37.

Gilkerson, L., Gorski, P. A., & Panitz, P. (1990). Hospital-based intervention for preterm infants and their families. In S. J. Meisels & J. P. Shonkoff (Eds.), *Handbook of early childhood intervention.* New York: Cambridge University Press (pp. 445–468).

Glass, R. P., & Wolf, L. S. (1994). A global perspective on feeding assessment in the neonatal intensive care unit. *The American Journal of Occupational Therapy, 48,* 514–526.

Goldberg, S., Corter, C., Lojkasek, M., & Minde, K. (1990). Prediction of behavior problems in 4 year olds born prematurely. *Development and Psychopathology, 2,* 15–30.

Gorski, P. A., Hole, W. T., Hole, C. H., & Martin, J. A. (1983). Direct recording of premature infants and nursery care. *Pediatrics, 72,* 198–202.

Gorski, P. A., Hole, W. T., Leonard, C. H., & Martin, J. A. (1983). Direct computer recording of premature infants and nursery care: Distress following two interventions. *Pediatrics, 72,* 198–202.

Gottfried, A. W., & Gaiter, J. L. (1985). *Infant stress under intensive care: Environmental neonatology.* Baltimore: University Park Press.

Hasselmeyer, E. G. (1964). The premature neonate's response to handling. *American Nurses' Association, 11,* 15–24.

Hayes, M. S., & Ensher, G. L. (1994). Intervening in intensive care nurseries. In G. L. Ensher & D. A. Clark (Eds.), *Newborns at risk: Medical care and psychoeducational intervention* (pp. 227–248). Rockville, MD: Aspen Publishers.

Heriza, C. B., & Sweeney, J. K. (1990). Effects of NICU intervention on preterm infants: Part 1—Implications for neonatal practice. *Infant and Young Children, 2,* 31–47.

Jorgenson, K. M. (1993). *Developmental care of the preterm infant: A concise overview.* Boston: Children's Medical Ventures.

Katz, V. (1971). Auditory stimulation and developmental behavior of the premature infant. *Nursing Research, 20,* 196–201.

Kilgo, J., Holder-Brown, L., Johnson, L. J., & Cook, M. J. (1988). An examination of the effects of tactile-kinesthetic stimulation on the development of preterm infants. *Journal of the Division for Early Childhood, 12,* 320–327.

Kimble, C., & Dempsey, J. (1992). Nonnutritive sucking: Adaptation and health for the neonate. *Neonatal Network, 11,* 29–33.

Klein, N., Hack, M., Gallagher, J., & Fanaroff, A. A. (1985). Preschool performance of children with normal intelligence who were very low birthweight infants. *Pediatrics, 75,* 531–537.

Kling, P. (1989). Nursing interventions to decrease the risk of periventricular/intraventricular hemorrhage. *Journal of Obstetrics, Gynecologic, and Neonatal Nursing, 18,* 457–464.

Kopp, C. B. (1983). Risk factors in development. In P. H. Mussen (Series Ed.), *Handbook of child psychiatry* (4th ed., Vol. 2). In J. J. Campos & M. Haith (Eds.), *Infancy and developmental psychobiology* (pp. 1081–1088). New York: Wiley.

Korner, A. F., Guilleminault, C., Van den Hood, M. D., & Baldwin, R. B. (1978). Reduction of sleep apnea and bradycardia in preterm infants on oscillating water beds: A controlled polygraphic study. *Pediatrics, 61,* 28–534.

Korner, A. F., Kraemer, H. C., Haffner, M. E., & Cosper, L. M. (1975). Effects of water bed flotation on premature infants: A pilot study. *Pediatrics, 56,* 361-367.

Korner, A. F., Ruppel, E. M., & Rho, J. M. (1982). Effects of water beds on the sleep and motility of Theophylline-treated preterm infants. *Pediatrics, 70,* 864–869.

Korner, A. F., Schneider, P., & Forest, T. (1983). Effects of vestibular-proprioceptive stimulation on the neurobehavioral development of preterm infants: A pilot study. *Neuropediatrics, 14,* 170–175.

Kramer, L. I., & Pierpont, M. E. (1976). Rocking waterbeds and auditory stimuli to enhance growth of preterm infants. *Journal of Pediatrics, 88,* 297–299.

Kramer, M., Chamorro, I., Green, D., & Knudtson, F. (1975). Extra tactile stimulation of the premature infant. *Nursing Research, 24*, 324–334.

Kuhn, C. M., Schanberg, S. M., Field, T., Symanski, R., Zimmerman, E., Scafidi, F., & Roberts, J. (1991). Tactile-kinesthetic stimulation effects on sympathetic and adrenocortical function in preterm infants. *Journal of Pediatrics, 119*, 434–440.

Laine, A. M. (1987). Kangaroo care in Turker's University Hospital Pediatric Clinic. *Katiloleht, 92*, 171–176.

Lefrak-Okikawa, L., & Lund, C. H. (1993). Nursing practice in the neonatal intensive care unit. In M. H. Klaus & A. A. Fanaroff (Eds.), *Care of the high-risk neonate* (pp. 212–227). Philadelphia: W. B. Saunders.

Leib, S. A., Benfield, G., & Guidubaldi, J. (1980). Effect of early intervention and stimulation of the preterm infant. *Pediatrics, 66*, 63–89.

Levine, S. (1962). The psychophysiological effects of infantile stimulation. In E. Bliss (Ed.), *Roots of behavior: Genetics, instinct and socialization in animal behavior* (pp. 235–245). New York: Hoeber.

Long, J. G., Phillips, A. C. S., & Lucey, J. F. (1980). Excessive handling as a cause of hypoxemia. *Pediatrics, 65*, 203–207.

Ludington, A. M. (1990). Energy conservation during skin-to-skin contact between premature infants and their mothers. *Heart and Lung, 19*, 445–451.

Masi, W. (1979). Supplemental stimulation of the premature infant. T. M. Field (Ed.), *Infants born at risk* (pp. 367–387). New York: S. P. Medical and Scientific Books.

McCormick, M. C. (1989). Long-term follow-up of infants discharged from neonatal intensive care units. *Journal of the American Medical Association, 261*, 24–31.

Measel, C. P., & Anderson, G. C. (1979). Non-nutritive sucking during tube feeding: Effect on clinical course in premature infants. *Journal of Obstetrics, Gyneologic, and Neonatal Nursing, 8*, 265–272.

Meier, P. (1993, July). *Breast-feeding the high-risk neonate:* Part I. Paper presented at Troubled Beginnings: Help for the Vulnerable Infant and Family in the Hospital and Community, Seattle, WA.

Miller, M. Q., & Hurst, M. Q. (1994). Neurobehavioral assessment of high-risk infants in neonatal intensive care. *The American Journal of Occupational Therapy, 48*, 506–513.

Morrow, C. J., Field, T. M., Scafidi, F. A., Roberts, J., Eisen, L., Larson, S. K., Hogan, A. E., & Bandstra, E. S. (1991). Differential effects of message and heelstick procedure on transcutaneous oxygen tension in preterm neonates. *Infant Behavior and Development, 14*, 397–414.

Murdoch, D. R., & Darlow, B. A. (1984). Handling during neonatal intensive care. *Archives of Disease in Childhood, 59*, 957–961.

Neal, M. (1968). Vestibular stimulation and the development behavior of the small premature infant. *Nursing Research Report, 3*, 1–5.

Neal, M. V. (1977). Vestibular stimulation and development of the small premature infant. *Communicating Nursing Research, 8*, 291–303.

Norris, S., Campbell, L., & Brenkhert, S. (1982). Nursing procedures and alterations in transcutaneous oxygen tension in premature infants. *Nursing Research, 31*, 330–333.

Pelletier, J. M., Short, M. A., & Nelson, D. L. (1985). Immediate effects of waterbed flotation on approach and avoidance behaviors of premature infants. *Physical and Occupational Therapy in Pediatrics, 5*, 81–92.

Pickler, R. H., & Frankel, H. (1995). The effect of non-nutritive sucking on preterm infants' behavioral organization and feeding performance. *Neonatal Network, 14*, 83.

Pickler, R. H., & Terrell, B. V. (1994). Nonnutritive sucking and necrotizing enerocolitis. *Neonatal Network, 13*, 15–18.

Powell, L. F. (1974). The effect of extra stimulation and maternal involvement on the development of low birthweight infants and on maternal behavior. *Child Development, 45*, 106–113.

Resnick, M. B., Armstrong, S., & Carter, R. L. (1988). Developmental intervention program for high-risk premature infants: Effects on development and parent-infant interactions. *Journal of Developmental and Behavioral Pediatrics, 9*, 73–78.

Rose, S. A., Schmidt, K., Riese, M. L., & Bridger, W. H. (1980). Effects of prematurity and early intervention on responsivity to tactical stimuli: A comparison of preterm and full-term infants. *Child Development, 51*, 416–425.

Ross, E. F. (1984). Review and critique of research on the use of tactile and kinesthetic stimilation with premature infants. *Physical & Occupational Therapy in Pediatrics, 4*, 35–49.

Scafidi, F. A., Field, T., & Schanberg, S. M. (1993). Factors that predict which preterm infants benefit most from message therapy. *Journal of Developmental and Behavioral Pediatrics, 14*, 176–180.

Scafidi, F., Field, T. M., Schanberg, S. M., Bauer, C. R., Vega-Lahr, N., Garcia, R., Poirier, J., Nystrom, G., & Kuhn, C. M. (1986). Effects of tactile/kinesthetic stimulation on the clinical course and sleep/wake behavior of preterm neonates. *Infant Behavior and Development, 9*, 91–105.

Scarr-Salpatek, S., & Williams, M. I. (1973). The effects of early stimulation on low birthweight infants. *Child Development, 44*, 94–101.

Segal, M. V. (1972). Cardiac responsivity to auditory stimulation in preterm infants. *Nursing Research, 21*, 15–19.

Solkoff, N., Jaffee, S., Weintraub, D., & Blase, B. (1969). Effects of handling on the subsequent development of premature infants. *Developmental Psychology, 1*, 765–786.

Solkoff, N., & Matuszak, D. (1975). Tactile stimulation and behavioral development among low-birthweight infants. *Child Psychiatry and Human Development, 6*, 33–37.

Thurman, S. K. (1993). Intervention in the neonatal intensive care unit. In W. Brown, S. K. Thurman, & L. F. Pearl (Eds.), *Family centered early intervention with infants and toddlers: Innovative cross-disciplinary approaches* (pp 173–209). Baltimore: Paul H. Brookes.

Tuck, S. J., Monin, P., Duvivier, C., May, T., & Vert, P. (1982). Effect of a rocking bed on apnoea of prematurity. *Archives of Disease in Childhood, 57*, 475–477.

Vohr, B. R. (1991). Preterm cognitive development: Biologic and environmental influences. *Infants and Young Children, 3*, 20–29.

White, J. L., & LaBarbar, R. C. (1976). The effects of tactile and kinesthetic stimulation on neonatal development in the premature infant. *Developmental Psychobiology, 6*, 569–577.

Whitelaw, A. (1990). Kangaroo baby care: Just a nice experience or an important advance for preterm infants? *Pediatrics, 85*, 604–605.

Whitelaw, A., Heisterkamp, G., Sleath, K., Acolet, D., & Richards, M. (1988). Skin-to-skin contact for very low birth weight infants and their mothers. *Achives Disease Childhood, 63*, 1377–1380.

Whitelaw, A., & Sleath, K. (1985). Myth of the marsupial mother: Home care for very low birth weight infants in Bogota, Colombia. *Lancet, 1*, 1206–1208.

Woodson, R., Drinkwin, J., & Hamilton, C. (1985). Effects of non nutritive sucking on state and activity: Term-preterm comparisons. *Infant Behavior and Development, 8*, 435–441.

■ CHAPTER 6
Developmental Interventions

> *If this child thrives under your devoted*
> *care, may its face shine. May it uproot*
> *the nightshade bushes with its brushing*
> *thigh. May it not become ill.*
> (West African prayer to protect the newborn,
> Dunham et al., 1991)

Once upon a time, in a world filled with wonderful machines there lived a growing fetus. This little human did not know about the wonderful machines because she was inside of her mother's uterus and there were no machines there. She was waiting for the wonderful promise of her new body. Then she was born too soon. Her body was not finished but the machines were there to help. The machines helped her breathe, they helped nourish her. Sometimes those things that helped her live hurt her. Her new eyes were not finished but they tried to see. She saw too many things which also made it hard to learn what was what. So she closed her eyes. The machines gave great noises for grownup ears, but her ears were new and tender and the noise was too loud. She was very tired. Many hands touched her. Sometimes a touch was nice and soft but many times it was sharp and painful. She tried but could not learn when a gentle touch would come; she would cry with every touch. She tried to sleep but the machines only let her sleep when they were ready. Her new brain learned the ways of the machines. Then one day her body was strong and the machines left. She cried in the quiet. She cried with the feel of food on her lips because she knew only plastic. A different touch now came with gentle sounds and big faces. It was so much to learn and she was tired. She looked away. She was confused because she knew only the language of machines. She looked away. She had learned to look away from the machines when she was tired, but the big faces were not machines and they did not understand. They were sad when she looked away. Her body was strong now but her brain had learned the wrong language. No one had taught her the language of people.

■ INTRODUCTION

Advances in neonatal medical technology and care have progressed more rapidly than any other medical field (Aumann, 1988). Technical miracles are common and have resulted, for example, in the survival of infants born as early as 23 weeks gestation and weighing as little as 454 grams (1 pound). Such very premature infants demand months of hospitalization involving ventilators and life-supporting intravenous fluids. In these situations, NICUs emphasize highly technical care and often pay only scant attention to developmentally supported interventions. For example, overhead lights often remain at full power to help caregivers see the patient and the equipment. This is a response to the technological aspects of the infant's care. If, however, the developmental aspects were part of that care plan, lights would be dimmed in an attempt to provide infants with a normal diurnal cycle.

Caregivers caught up in the demands of high technology often wait until the infant has been weaned from technical support before incorporating formal developmental interventions into care plans. Developmental interventions, however, can begin with any infant's admission to the intensive care nursery. Many health care providers unknowingly already incorporate many aspects of developmental interventions into their routine care. Such actions as repositioning the infant or simply touching the infant in a gentle manner are examples of developmental interventions.

Fortunately, many intensive care units are now paying greater attention to the contributions of developmentally based interventions. This chapter highlights what we have learned. The first section of the chapter describes the evolution of developmentally supportive care in NICUs. Then questions basic to the concept of developmental interventions are addressed. For example, developmental interventions will be explored within the context of routine care for the infant in the NICU. Finally, developmental interventions appropriate for specific gestational age groups are described, and interventions that parents and caregivers can use are addressed.

■ THE NICU: MOVING TOWARD INDIVIDUALIZED CARE

A brief examination of the fairly recent past will provide a picture of how NICUs developed their strong technological emphasis. The earliest hospitals in the United States were adult care facilities that originated in the mid 1800s in response to two major historical events (Rosenberg, 1987). First, when people flocked to the cities in pursuit of the many jobs created by the Industrial Revolution, they often came without the grandmothers, mothers, aunts, sisters, or wives who had been responsible for the family's health needs. When the new city dwellers became ill, they were often too far from their rural homes to be helped by the traditional family unit. They had no place to go for health care. Over time community leaders recognized the need for facilities to care for ill workers, if only to return them expediently to their jobs. Hospitals were built to realize this business goal.

Second, the Civil War and World War I resulted in large numbers of injured soldiers requiring organized care to regain their health (Rosenberg, 1987). The sooner these soldiers were able to return to the battle, the greater the military advantage. Military hospitals were formed based on this strategic goal.

Although different in goals, both types of hospitals focused on returning ill men and women to health. Before long hospitals became accepted replacements for the health care that had been given within the family (Rosenberg, 1987). This shift fostered an emotional distancing between the patient and the health care provider. Basically, hospital care became the care of strangers by strangers.

As hospitals grew and became more sophisticated so did medical technology. Soon areas of the hospitals that were centers for advanced technology became known as intensive care units. These units were designed to care for adult patients with acute illness. The units provided the most technologically advanced care possible and, when patients improved sufficiently, the intensive care units returned patients to the less intensive ward for recuperation. The adult hospital patients' only task was to get better. There was little need to provide an environment that also was concerned about patients' growth and development.

Although advances in neonatal medical technology have progressed more rapidly than advances in other medical fields (Aumann, 1988), medical understanding of the newborn in the mid 1800s and early 1900s was not sophisticated by modern standards. The major advancement in neonatal medical technology during the mid 1800s and early 1900s was understanding the importance of providing warmth and nourishment for the premature infant. In the late 1800s Etienne Tarnier, a French physician, invented the incubator and gavage feedings (Lyons, 1985). For premature infants, too small and weak to maintain body temperature or nutritive sucking, this advancement was essential for survival. But even as late as 1963, medical technology was not yet sophisticated enough to solve the respiratory problems of premature infants of 33 weeks gestation. For example, in 1963 Patrick Kennedy, the son of the late President John

F. Kennedy, was born at 33 weeks gestation and died 3 days later of respiratory complication (Lyons, 1985). Today, with the advent of surfactant and pressure ventilatory support, an infant of 33 weeks gestation would have an excellent chance for survival.

In the mid 1950s neonatal intensive care units were modeled after adult intensive care units. NICUs had the latest technology, a centralized location, and skilled health care providers. As in adult intensive care units, the focus of NICU care was to return the neonate to health. This occurred even though premature infants were not ill in the same sense that adult patients were ill. Infants, for example, were often quite stable and healthy, requiring minimal technical support to gain enough weight for discharge home.

As NICU caregivers became more aware of differences between premature infants and ill adults, concern for neonates' growth and development began to emerge. Professionals became sensitive to the impact of their technology on NICU infants' growth and development. Developmentally supportive care began to be considered an important component of routine treatment in the neonatal unit. This led many NICU environments to become more developmentally appropriate. Today, progressive NICUs incorporate developmental interventions into infants' routine care.

The new interest in developmental interventions led to research on the effects of the NICU environment on infant behaviors as well as the effects of the infant's separation from the family. Modern research revealed that the NICU environment can be restructured to offer decreased stress from lighting, noise, and activity without compromising the life saving care necessary (Als, 1986; Anderson, 1986; Mann, Haddow, Stokes, Goodley, & Rutter, 1986). Velasco-Whetsell, Evans, and Wang (1992) found that the stress of physical care such as endotracheal suctioning can be reduced with touch and containment procedures. Yoos (1989) has shown ways to support parenting preterm infants even in the technical NICU environment.

Ignoring the benefits of developmental interventions assumes infants are only hospitalized for physiological needs. Nothing could be further from the truth. Infants strive for normal growth and development in the face of enormous physiological needs. A central task of NICU caregivers is to provide infants with appropriate opportunities to grow and develop even within the highly technical NICU environment. In the next section we will more closely examine developmental interventions.

■ DEVELOPMENTAL INTERVENTIONS

What Are Developmental Interventions?

Development refers to the normal growth and maturation of an infant. Intervention is care, tailored to a preterm or full-term infant's specific developmental stage. For example, when a mother turns off the lights to let her newborn sleep in a quiet, dark room she is using a developmental intervention. Infants naturally develop circadian rhythms which foster quiet sleep times and active alert times. The mother enhances this developing circadian rhythm by intervening with an environment conducive to the infant's desire to sleep. When a caregiver swaddles a premature infant after an invasive procedure such as heelstick blood drawing, a developmental intervention is taking place. The caregiver is intervening with swaddling and supporting the infant's developing ability to self-comfort. Placing infants of similar developmental stages together is another example of an intervention that can help support the infants' developmental progress. The clustering of infants of similar developmental stages allows caregivers greater ease in maintaining quiet times with reduced noise and lighting. A stable growing premature infant will not benefit from the noise, high lighting, and acute activity surrounding a newly admitted infant in the next bedspace.

Developmental interventions can be protective actions such as covering an isolette with a blanket to protect an infant from overhead lighting. Another protective developmental intervention is clustering routine care to provide frequent episodes of rest between the care (Als et al., 1994). For example, if the infant can tolerate one clustered episode of contact including vital signs, blood drawing, and diagnostic testing, a rest period devoid of contact can follow. It is important to assess the infant frequently during clustered care to determine tolerance of the activity. If signs indicate the infant is having difficulty tolerating the activity, an appropriate developmental intervention would be to stop the clustered care and allow the infant to recover.

Developmental interventions can also stimulate infants. Speaking softly to the infant provides auditory stimuli. Positioning the infant with blanket roll support provides tactile stimulation. Once again, however, an intervention should be tailored to the specific infant's developmental status.

Developmental interventions do not need to be complex. They can be protective and they can stimulate. Routine care in an intensive care nursery includes many aspects of developmental care. In fact NICU health care providers perform many developmental interventions without consciously knowing this is what they are doing. Expert caregivers, however, knowingly match interventions with the developmental status of each infant. This matching requires an understanding of the infant's developmental progression. Using a developmental model is a helpful way to understand and assess an infant's developmental status.

One important model of development used with the preterm infant is the one created by Als in the synactive theory of development. This model examines the behavioral developmental progression of preterm infants through four interactive subsystems which include the physiologic subsystem, the motoric subsystem, attentional/interactive subsystem, and the behavioral states (Als, 1986). The interaction of these subsystems is mutually interdependent. When one subsystem is disrupted, the normal progression of development in the other subsystems is delayed. The maturation of each subsystem supports interactions among and between the other subsystems. In turn, this creates stability within the system as a whole and development progresses. For example, the infant's muscle control, part of the motor subsystem, develops in a caudocephalal direction (Creger & Browne, 1989). This means that the infant will normally gain leg muscle control before arm muscle control. The infant will find boundaries by stretching out legs before finding comfort by moving hands to mouth. An improvement in the control of the lower extremities can be seen by 29–30 weeks post-conceptual age while the upper extremities gain this type of muscle control 2–4 weeks later (Creger & Browne, 1989). Understanding this model helps the NICU caregiver tailor interventions specific for the developmental status of this 29–30 week infant.

How Can Developmental Intervention Be Matched to Each Infant?

Matching developmental intervention with an infant's developmental status is often difficult. VandenBerg (1985) refers to this difficulty when she states "Many intervention approaches seek to reduce the negative effects of the NICU by increasing the infant's sensory experience. However, the first systematic exploration of sensory experiences in the NICU concluded that infants suffer from an inappropriate pattern rather than an inadequate amount of stimulation" (p. 33). To prevent an inappropriate pattern from occurring, it is essential to assess the infant before initiating an intervention. Through assessment, the NICU caregiver determines whether the infant is developmentally ready for the specific intervention (White-Traut, Nelson, Burns, & Cunningham, 1994).

Let us examine the activity of a NICU nurse to illustrate the process of matching an intervention to infant developmental status.

Nurse Smith is taking care of an infant who is 33 weeks gestational age, weighing 2200 grams. It is time for this infant's feeding. It would be developmentally inappropriate for Nurse Smith to feed this infant a peanut butter sandwich. Even the inexperienced caregiver would recognize the futility of such a feeding. What is the developmentally appropriate type of feeding for this infant? An infant of 33 weeks gestational age should be mature enough to coordinate suck and swallow and take nipple feedings. However, this specific infant may not be able to coordinate suck and swallow and may need oralgastric tube feedings. After Nurse Smith assesses this infant's abilities, she chooses the type of feeding. She is matching the intervention to the infant's developmental status.

Caregivers who understand the behaviors typical of different gestational ages can assess infants with these basic expectations in mind. The comparison between what the infant can do and what the infant should be able to do helps describe the infant's capabilities. It is only when the infant's capabilities are recognized that there can be a match between intervention and infant developmental status.

Matching developmental interventions and infant capabilities can also occur when comforting an infant. Some would argue that tailoring comforting measures to the infant is too time consuming to use efficiently within the busy pace of the NICU. They would say it is easier to allow an infant to cry itself to sleep than to stand at the bedside holding a nonnutritive pacifier in place while the infant calms. However, allowing the infant to calm down using its ability to suck on a pacifier helps the infant experience the normal progression toward self-comfort. The infant allowed to cry and fuss without intervention becomes more and more disorganized. More time is then consumed returning the infant to a stable state. The point is to intervene before the infant reaches the endpoint of disorganization. Intervention at this time is developmentally appropriate. If no one intervenes and the infant progresses to vomiting, apnea, desaturation, and self-extubation, time will be consumed anyway to attend to the infant's physical needs. To conserve time and offer optimal care, an expert caregiver will assess the infant and rapidly intervene with comforting measures matched to the infant's developmental status.

When Can Developmental Interventions Begin?

The answer to this question lies in appreciating each infant's developmental status and developmental needs. Often the most appropriate developmental intervention is to not touch the infant. Caregivers may have difficulty understanding that it appropriate not to touch a patient, especially when the hospital is viewed as an environment where hands-on care is expected. For example, an infant of 23 weeks gestation can tolerate very little outside stimulation without physiological decompensation. Knowing this, caregivers may choose to assess the infant simply by looking while not touching the infant at all. The infant's vital signs such as heart rate may be obtained from the cardiac monitor. Taking the heart rate in this fashion obviates the need to touch the infant's chest with a stethoscope. Endotracheal tube suctioning for this infant may be deferred and done only when clinical parameters such as rising CO_2s, decreased chest movement, or diminished breath sounds indicate the need. Many NICUs today have minimal stimulation protocols based on the infant's very limited tolerance for stimuli.

NICU patients do not spend all of their lives in the life and death clutches of modern technology and medicine. An infant may rapidly reach a stable physiologic state that requires minimal equipment support. During this stable period, infants will quickly gain weight, learn to take nourishment orally, learn to adjust to the surrounding environment, and begin to adapt to caretaker interaction (Avery & Taeusch, 1984; Creger, 1993). Often caregivers incorporate developmental interventions only within the context of routine patient care. However, during stable periods, it is appropriate to begin providing infants with specific developmental interventions tailored to their skills (Burns, Cunningham, White-Traut, Silvestri, & Nelson, 1994).

A broad range of developmental stimuli is available for the growing infant. Caregivers can provide tactile and vestibular stimulation by holding or rocking the infant. They can talk to the infant and thereby provide auditory stimulation. Mobiles or bright toys can be placed around the infant to provide visual stimulation. Any intervention, whether protective or stimulating, should be preceeded by an understanding of the infant's developmental status, knowledge of the interventions appropriate for the infant's skill level, and a desire to match the two (Yecco, 1993). Later in this chapter, developmental interventions appropriate for specific gestational age groups will be discussed.

Developmental interventions should begin as soon as the infant is admitted to the NICU. Frequently the initial interventions limit touching the infant. Later, when the infant's developmental status matures, interventions may include providing the infant with age-appropriate stimuli such as holding or rocking the infant.

Who Is Responsible for Initiating Developmental Interventions?

Virtually anyone who touches the infant is responsible for assuring that the touch or other interventions match the infant's developmental status. Bedside caregivers and parents have a special responsibility in developmental interventions. Bedside caregivers have the most numerous infant contacts affording them many opportunities to initiate various interventions. In fact, research literature has reported NICU infants have over 200 contacts daily. NICU nurses are responsible for 86% of these contacts (Medoff-Cooper, 1988; Peters, 1992).

Bedside caregivers may be forced to handle infants frequently for medical procedures, but to do so without regard for the infant's skill at coping with touch is unconscionable. Second, in their role as a patient advocate, the caregivers are instrumental in directing the type and frequency of interaction between other professionals and the infant. Parents have the greatest personal investment in the infant and frequently initiate developmental interventions to generate infant interaction. The skilled parent will need to understand the infant's developmental status, have knowledge of interventions appropriate for the infant's skill level, and be able to match the two. The bedside caregiver can help facilitate parents in this quest.

What Steps Are Necessary To Match and Implement Developmental Interventions?

Several steps are essential for successfully implementing matched developmental interventions. The first step is to assess the infants' developmental status, stress signs, and skill at self-comfort. The second step is to recognize how much stimulation the infant can tolerate or cannot tolerate. The third step is to be aware of the infant's medical status and immediate environmental input. The fourth step is to decide on an intervention based on the information obtained from the first three steps.

Looking at a developmental intervention for a 30-week gestational age infant will illustrate this process. This process will seem ponderous. However, in reality, this thought process occurs rapidly and automatically for expert caregivers. The decisions are predicated by:

■ an understanding of the infant's developmental status
■ assessment of the infant's activities and the outcomes of these activities
■ skill in matching interventions to the infant and supporting the infant's developing capabilities.

First the NICU caregiver assesses the infant's muscle tone comparing the tone to that expected from a typical infant of 30 weeks. The caregiver sees the infant is in active sleep with rapid eye movement behind closed lids and sucking motions of the mouth. At this moment the infant is showing no signs of stress. The infant has snuggled against the isolette wall exhibiting some skill at self-comfort by using developing muscle tone to move around and find boundaries. Als' Synactive Theory predicts that this infant's muscle control will not be not fully developed, and this limited development will affect stability of state organization in the face of external stimulation (Als, 1982). Therefore, the NICU caregiver recognizes this infant may be able to tolerate being touched but may not tolerate more invasive procedures such as heelstick blood sampling.

The infant's medical status, however, requires blood sampling by heelstick for electrolyte analysis. When the blood work is drawn, the infant reacts by desaturating as evidenced by a drop in pulse oximetry. The physiologic subsystem has been disrupted; the infant becomes hypoxic, tachycardic, and tachypneic. To stabilize this disruption the infant seeks self-comforting measures, part of the state organization subsystem. Self-comforting measures include bringing hands to mouth and seeking boundaries, but because the infant's muscle control is not yet fully developed, the infant cannot achieve these goals. The state organization subsystem is affected by the limited development of the motoric system.

Lacking sufficient self-comforting abilities, the infant has difficulty stabilizing physiological responses to the painful heelstick. If the caregiver does not intervene, the infant's physiologic instability continues. The pulse oximeter continues to drop, the infant vomits, and becomes completely hypotonic. The caregiver, however, is an expert and intervenes immediately. This infant has shown initial attempts at self-comforting seeking boundaries, so the caregiver chooses to continue these attempts. The infant's arms are brought to midline and flexed so that the hands are close to the mouth. The caregiver then places her hands around the infant, with one hand supporting the lower extremities and the other hand cupping the head, offering the infant boundaries. The infant is held in this position until quiet and exhibiting normal pulse oximeter values. The developmental intervention has included helping the infant self-comfort and regain a midline flexed position (see Figure 6–1).

It is interesting to note that adults also seek self-comfort in a midline, flexed position, such as resting hands close to the face. Take a moment and look at your position right now. Are your hands as far away from your face as possible and are your arms and legs fully stretched out? Unlikely. It is likely you are resting with your hand on your chin or perhaps your hand is against your forehead. This flexion and midline positioning is a comfort to us as well as to the infant.

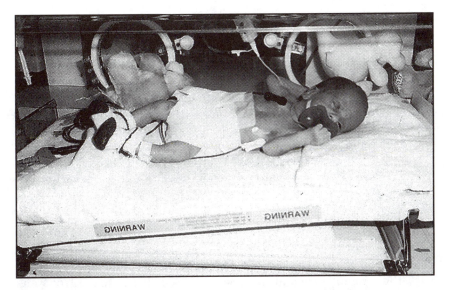

FIGURE 6–1. Infant flexed and attempting self-regulation. (Photograph courtesy of Children's Hospital of Buffalo Department of Medical Photography.)

Caregiver-Matched Intervention

What might an expert caregiver be thinking or how might the expert reach decisions in the above example? Remember the infant of 30 weeks gestation has just experienced an invasive medical procedure. The caregiver might think:

1. I see the infant is in active sleep and has found boundaries by snuggling against the isolette wall.
2. I know this infant will not tolerate much external stimuli.
3. I must obtain a blood sample by heelstick in order to manage this infant's IV fluids correctly. Since the infant is in active sleep, now would be a good time to obtain the blood work. I expect the stimuli of the heelstick to disrupt the infant's sleep state.
4. After obtaining the heelstick sample, I see the infant cry, desaturate, and vomit. I can clean the infant but I also want to leave this infant in a quiet state. I know a quiet state is the optimal state for infant growth. I have already

seen this infant seek her own boundaries by snuggling against the isolette. since infants become quiet when given boundaries and containment, I will try to match this technique to this infant. I also know she will have more difficulty getting her hands to her mouth because of her gestational age. When I position her, I will take care to position her arms in a flexed manner with her hands nestled by her mouth. I will then place my hands around her, with one hand supporting her lower extremities and the other hand cupping her head. I will hold her until she is quiet. This intervention may delay my departure from her bedside but it is necessary to help her maintain a quiet, restful state.

Parent-Matched Intervention

It is important to support parents' understanding of their infant's developmental status so they too will be able to match interventions with their infant's capabilities (Belsky, 1984; Brazleton, 1975; Kenner & Lott, 1990; Pridham, 1993). But why burden parents with developmental information about their infant if they are not going to take, for example, an infant of 25 weeks gestation home for several months? Don't parents have enough to worry about already?

Dealing with the crisis of a premature infant or an infant sick enough to need intensive care can be devastating for parents (Miles, 1989; Yoos, 1989). Studies indicate the highest stress for mothers of these infants is the change in their parental role followed by the sights and sounds of the unit (Affonso et al., 1992; Miles, 1989; Yoos, 1989).

When health care professionals help parents match appropriate interventions to their infant's developmental capabilities, they are supporting the development of parenting skills (Cusson & Lee, 1993). When parents provide skilled parenting to their infant their role is reinforced. The new mother of a 23-week gestation infant may have fantasized about holding her infant and gazing into his eyes. It is important for this mother to understand that her infant is not developmentally ready to see. Her infant's eyes are still fused. However, she can be supported to use the visiting hours to sit by her infant's bedside and get to know her infant simply by looking at him. She can begin to recognize the physical characteristics that make her infant unique. Often parents are the first ones to recognize their infant's emerging developmental skills. This new mother may be, for example, the one to tell the nurse that her infant can now open his eyes.

Parents, with a little direction from health care professionals, can be a valuable resource to help ameliorate the impact of the NICU environment on their infants. For example, parents of an infant of 32 weeks gestation can be encouraged to make tapes of themselves reading nursery stories and bring these tapes to the NICU to play for their infant. Instead of listening to alarms, their infant listens to their voices.

Parents can also be encouraged to comfort their infants following invasive procedures such as vital signs or heelsticks. They may need directions at first to understand exactly what comforting interventions are appropriate to their infant's developmental status. Once the parents begin to know their infant's unique characteristics and developmental status, they become valuable resources in tailoring care for their infant. Within the highly technical world of the intensive care nursery, parents acting as advocates for their infant can lend an air of humanity to the unit.

■ IMPLEMENTING DEVELOPMENTAL INTERVENTIONS

The premature infant enters the world with certain potential to develop self-comforting actions, maintain alert states that foster interaction, and develop skills to cope with their environment. These emerging skills are the developmental status that a caregiver assesses prior to initiating developmental interventions. These skills, evident when the infant responds to **tactile**, **visual**, and **auditory** stimuli change as infants grow and develop. This section examines premature infant's responses within these three areas of stimuli. Developmental intervention for various gestational age groups are suggested.

Tactile Stimulation

Infants as early as 23 weeks gestation are born with functioning tactile and vestibular systems (Avery & Taeusch, 1984; Beachy & Deacon, 1993; Creger & Browne, 1989; Field, 1990). The vestibular system includes the end-organs of the inner ear and neuron connections between the inner ear and the brain (Creger & Browne, 1989; Langman, 1991). This system is responsible for maintaining equilibrium, directing eye gaze, and maintaining a plane of vision dependent upon head position (Creger & Browne, 1989). When newborn infants with an intact central nervous system are moved from side to side in a horizontal plane, their eyes will move in a direction opposite of their body in order to maintain a constant point of focus (Field, 1990).

The tactile system is responsible for the infant's neurological awareness of the environment. Neonatal reflexive behaviors are elicited responses to tactile stimulation. At 28 weeks gestation, for example, infants will grasp an item placed in their hand (palmer reflex) (see Figure 6–2) and turn their head toward a touch on the cheek (rooting reflex) (Avery & Taeusch, 1984; Creger & Browne, 1989).

Developmentally supportive interventions involving the tactile and vestibular systems, include using:

- soft surfaces such as sheep skin or cotton velour blankets
- water or oscillating mattresses
- containment surfaces provided by blanket rolls
- slow, gentle changes of position
- warmed surfaces

Some of these interventions can be implemented in the infant's routine care. Each touch and position change can include a developmental intervention. Because positioning and handling infants is such a large part of neonatal caregiving, this portion of tactile stimulation will be addressed separately.

Positioning and Handling

Handling and positioning an infant provides one of the first opportunities for caregivers to use developmental interventions. The first question caregivers must ask is:

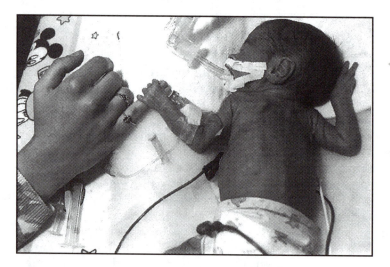

FIGURE 6–2. A preterm infant holds his mother's finger. (Photograph courtesy of Children's Hospital of Buffalo Department of Medical Photography.)

Is this infant too fragile to tolerate even being touched? If the answer to this question is "yes," limit touching. Consider interventions such as:

■ obtaining vital signs from the cardio-respiratory monitor instead of touching the infant.

■ limiting suctioning, for example, removing secretions of the endotracheal tube to times when auscultation (listening with a stethoscope) of the infant's chest indicates an increase in pulmonary secretions or blood gas parameters indicate a rising CO_2.

■ limiting heelstick blood drawing to a minimum.

■ limiting optional physical exams.

■ limiting any unnecessary handling of the infant.

If an infant tolerates being touched, the question for the caregiver to ask is:

Is this a good time for the infant to be touched and handled? Some caregivers feel the actual handling and positioning of an infant is a process without great developmental significance. They would argue (1) that each infant is touched so frequently during hospitalization that it is unreasonable to worry about the infant's developmental state before each contact, and (2) tactile stimuli is not as significant as visual or auditory stimuli.

Studies have shown that appropriate handling and positioning of premature infants during invasive procedures, such as endotracheal tube suctioning, fosters the infant's return to a resting state (Velasco-Whetsell et al., 1992). If the goal is to provide infants with long periods of rest it is easy to see why appropriate positioning and handling is so significant.

When infants are in quiet sleep every attempt **not** to disturb them should be made. If handling can be reasonably delayed it should be delayed. It is very important for the infant in quiet sleep to be allowed to continue sleeping (Heriza & Sweeney, 1990; McMillen, Kok, Adamson, Deayton, & Nowak, 1991).

When infants are disorganized and crying, their interaction with the environment may be developmentally inappropriate. Appropriate positioning and handling of infants before and after painful procedures assists infants to return to a quiet alert state needed to foster growth and development. Appropriate positioning and handling of infants moves them back into a rest state. The following example illustrates developmental interventions using positioning and handling.

Nurse Terri is a day shift RNC caring for an infant whose status is fairly stable following post surgical repair of a tracheal-esophageal fistula. At 7 AM, she wakes the infant from quiet sleep for heelstick blood work. During and after the procedure, the infant becomes very agitated and cries vigorously. The nurse has been assigned an early break and needs to complete her morning assessments with this infant before leaving. She chooses to spend a full 10 minutes after the heelstick returning this infant to a quiet sleep state. The techniques she uses to comfort this infant are:

■ containing the infant's arms and legs followed by gentle rocking
■ swaddling the infant
■ offering the infant a pacifier for nonnutritive sucking
■ covering the crib with a blanket to protect the infant from the glare of the lights

Once the infant has returned to a quiet sleep, the nurse places a note on the infant's crib to advise other caregivers not to disturb the infant for at least 1 hour. Although the time used to comfort the infant may have delayed the nurse's break, the interventions were in the infant's best interests. Repositioning an infant rapidly may also cause the infant to be disorganized.

Anyone who has worked in a neonatal intensive care unit has witnessed what happens when a premature infant is handled rapidly. The infant responds with wild gyrations, arms and legs flailing, a wide-eyed look, and general disorganization (see Figure 6–3). If an infant is awake or in active sleep when repositioning occurs, the caregiver can proceed to touch and move the infant slowly and deliberately. This slow, deliberate handling is especially comforting for premature infants who lack the muscle tone to counteract the effects of gravity themselves during position changes.

Specific Positioning Interventions

Now let us look with more detail at some specific position interventions used to provide developmentally supportive care.

REPOSITIONING. To reposition the infant from supine to prone or from prone to supine, gently hold the infant's legs and arms against the infant's body. Use one hand to cup the infant's feet and gently bend the legs so the knees are positioned close to the infant's abdomen. Use your other hand to gently fold the infant's arms across the chest. Once contained, wait for several seconds for the infant to adjust before moving to the next step (see Figure 6–4). Gently rotate the infant 90°. Wait for several seconds, allowing the infant to adjust to this change in position before moving to the next step (see Figure

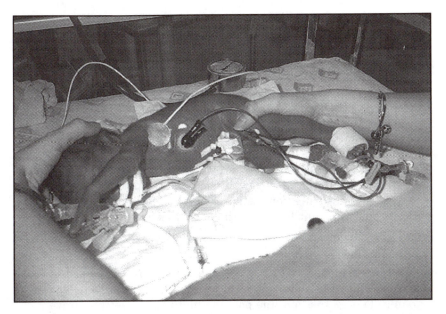

FIGURE 6–3. Infant response to brisk handling. (Photograph courtesy of Children's Hospital of Buffalo Department of Medical Photography.)

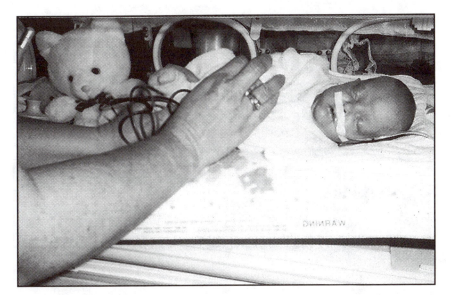

FIGURE 6–4. Initial step in repositioning infant. (Photograph courtesy of Children's Hospital of Buffalo Department of Medical Photography.)

6–5). Gently rotate the infant an additional 90° and wait for several seconds for the infant to adjust to this position (see Figure 6–6). Once the infant has been repositioned 180°, from supine to prone or from prone to supine, it is time to nest the infant. The term **nesting** refers to positioning the infant using blanket roll supports. Once the supports have been placed around the infant, the infant appears to be in a nest, hence the term.

SUPINE NESTING TECHNIQUES. Gently support the infant with blanket rolls so that the infant's shoulders are positioned slightly anterior. This positioning prevents posterior traction of the infant's shoulders and keeps the infant in good position for optimum movement of the diaphragm during ventilation. Snuggle blanket rolls close to the infant's left and right flanks so that the hips are kept close to a midline position. Maintain the arms and legs in a flexed position. Bring the infant's hands as close to the infant's face as possible.

PRONE NESTING TECHNIQUES. A small blanket roll is placed beneath the infant's hips allowing slight elevation of the infant's pelvis. Move the infant's legs to a midline position and flex the legs to prevent the thighs from lying flat against the mattress. Provide a blanket roll at the infant's feet to give a sense of containment. Flex the infant's arms

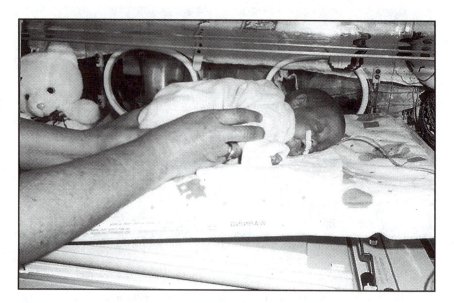

FIGURE 6–5. Second step in repositioning infant. (Photograph courtesy of Children's Hospital of Buffalo Department of Medical Photography.)

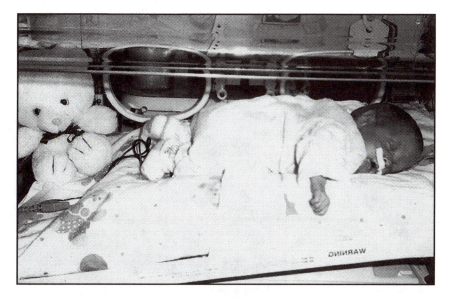

FIGURE 6–6. Infant ready to nest. (Photograph courtesy of Children's Hospital of Buffalo Department of Medical Photography.)

and move the hands as close to the face as possible. This promotes hands to mouth maneuvers. Alternate the position of the head so that the infant is not always facing one direction.

SIDE LYING NESTING TECHNIQUES. Gently place a long blanket roll above the infant's head and down the spine. The end of the roll can be placed either between the infant's legs to offer support for the thighs or at the infant's feet to offer a sense of containment. Flex the infant's legs at the knees and curl the blanket roll beneath the feet for support. Place a smaller roll along the infant's chest and abdomen to help maintain the side lying position. Move the arms around the anterior roll as if the infant is hugging the blanket and position the hands close to the infant's face (see Figure 6–7). It is equally important for NICU caregivers to use appropriate positioning and to share this information with the infant's parents. Parents need to learn how to comfort their infant using appropriate positioning and handling. Parents are often so eager to see their infant respond to them, they may use inappropriate interactions such as jostling the infant or flicking the infant's feet. If the infant becomes disorganized and irritable, parents become discouraged. Expert caregivers can help them use appropriate positioning and handling to comfort their infant.

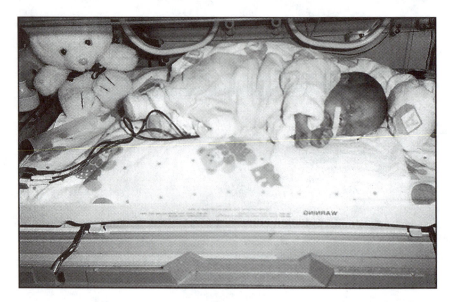

FIGURE 6–7. Side lying position. (Photograph courtesy of Children's Hospital of Buffalo Department of Medical Photography.)

When parents are comfortable interacting with and comforting their infant, they become valuable resources. This not only fosters parenting skills but also enhances parents' attachment with their infant. The following example illustrates ways that parents can be included in developmental care interventions:

> Nurse Russell is rushed and feels overworked. Baby Smith, a very active 32-week infant, has pulled out her oral-gastric tube, has wiggled out of her diaper, and cried so much that the cardiac monitor has alarmed falsely several times. Nurse Russell notices that Baby Smith is finally quiet. Then baby's father arrives for a visit. Immediately he goes to the infant's isolette, opens the portholes and tries to tickle the infant's feet in an attempt to awaken her. Disappointed that his baby shows so little response, Mr. Smith places his hand on the infant's back and gently shakes her. The baby awakens and starts crying.
>
> Nurse Russell stops and recognizes that intervention is necessary. She stops what she is doing, immediately goes to Mr. Smith and asks if he would like to see some comforting measures that his baby really seems to like. She demonstrates the calming technique of positioning a hand over the baby's head and cupping the baby's feet and legs. Mr. Smith then tries this while Nurse Russell talks him through the procedure, and after many attempts, Baby Smith finally quiets down. The

quieting of his baby reinforces Mr. Smith's actions, and he is content to stay at his baby's bedside with his hands gently providing comfort for his daughter.

Tactile stimulation is just one type of stimulation that has developmental consequences for premature infants (Thoman, Ingersull, & Acebo, 1991). Visual stimulation is another important developmental domain.

Visual Stimulation

The visual centers of the growing fetus are functionally complete by the 18th week of gestation (Langman, 1991). The eyelids, fused until the 23–25th week, continue to allow dark and light shades to penetrate the thin skin of the fetal lid (Witt, 1992). Infants delivered at 23 weeks gestation continue to sense the effect of bright light shining through their thin eyelids even though the lids are fused. Once the eyes open, an infant as young as 24 weeks gestational age can see objects within 8 to 10 inches of their face, provided the central nervous system is intact (Gardner, Garland, Merenstein, & Merenstein, 1989). This distance approximates the distance from an infant and a caregiver's face when the infant is nestled in the crook of the caregiver's arm.

Full-term infants have a visual preference for the human face and patterned objects (Field, 1990). Although full-term infants can discriminate color, their visual preference is for the contrast of bold black and white patterns, especially if the pattern resembles a human face (Gardner et al., 1989). Premature infants respond differently to visual stimuli than do full-term infants. At 30–32 weeks gestation, premature infants are only beginning to sustain focus on the contrast pattern that full-term infants prefer (Creger & Browne, 1989).

Studies of the effects of dimming lights and reducing noise in a day-night pattern for premature infants have shown dimming lights to be a major determinant in the emergence of a circadian sleep-wake pattern (McMillen et al., 1991). The advantage of a circadian sleep-wake pattern can include more restful sleep with increased weight gain due to the anabolic effect of quiet sleep and shorter feeding times, as well as more frequent active alert periods (Mann et al., 1986).

Because of their immature central nervous system, preterm infants may be able to tolerate only a single environmental stimuli at a time. For example, a 29-week infant may be able to tolerate only a brief visual stimuli such as the appearance of the mother's face. When this is the case, the person offering the interaction should look at the infant without additional tactile or auditory stimulation. As premature infants show increased tolerance, additional stimuli can be added to interactions. More complex visual stimuli can be used with older, stable preterm infants.

Ongoing assessment of the infant's reaction to visual stimuli is crucial when trying to provide appropriate stimuli without overloading the infant's tolerance capacity. It is especially important to assist parent's understanding of infant cues. Parents are often keenly aware of their infant's responses and can easily mistake a time-out signal such as gaze aversion for rejection.

Auditory Stimulation

The sensory portion of the auditory system in the human fetus is complete at 20 weeks gestation (Langman, 1991). The fetus in utero begins to hear and identify sounds before birth (Avery & Taeusch, 1984). The transmission portion of the auditory system has completed development by the 30th week of gestation (Creger & Browne, 1989). Even the very premature infant with an intact central nervous system will show response to sound. Full-term infants have been shown to prefer and to differentiate family voices from those of strangers (DeCasper & Fifer, 1983). Newborn infants also prefer high-pitched over lower-pitched voices (Freiberg, 1992).

Sound within the intensive care nursery is generated by much more than the human voice. While normal speaking voices have decibel levels of 50–60, the typical machine alarms and sounds within the NICU are much higher (Creger, 1993; Gardner et al., 1989). Just closing one or both incubator portholes can generate decibel levels of 130–140, and placing a bottle of formula on top of an isolette can generate noise at 96–117 decibels (Gardner et al., 1989). Awareness of both the excessive NICU noise levels and infants' ability to hear this noise helps caregivers actively protect the infant from unnecessary auditory stimuli.

■ SUGGESTIONS FOR PARENTS

The following section will address specific gestational ages of infants and describe developmental interventions appropriate to specific ages. These interventions can be implemented by both NICU caregivers and parents. If needed, NICU caregivers can teach parents to interact with their infant in ways that reflect the infant's developmental skills. It is important to emphasize that responses at specific gestational ages may vary from one infant to another. What is typical for one infant at 30 weeks may be typical for another infant at 32 weeks.

Infants 23 to 25 Weeks Gestation

Parents often try to use eye-to-eye contact to initiate their first interaction with their infant. This contact is reinforced when the infant fixes visually on the parent's face or turns his or her eyes in an attempt to follow the parent. However, such interaction is significantly limited with a very premature infant of 23 to 25 weeks gestation who may have fused eyelids. Even after they can open their eyes, the majority of very premature infants' time is spent in a drowsy sleep state. Although this sleep state is important for the growth and development of 23- to 25-week-old infant, parents can be discouraged by their limited interaction with their infant.

In situations like this, caregivers can explain to parents that their infant's eyelids may not be open at this early gestational age, but as the infant matures the eyelids will open. At this early age, an infant will not follow or "track" an item in their visual field. Parents should be encouraged to use this time to watch their infant. They can focus on becoming aware of their infant's unique physical qualities. If the infant is on a radiant warmer, position the infant with its face toward the parents. When possible, remove any eye coverings the infant may be wearing and turn off phototherapy lights so that the parents can see their infant's facial characteristics.

Although very preterm infants may not yet be able to visually focus on an object, they will be able to hear. In fact, at this early stage of development, any auditory stimulation may be overwhelming. Consequently, guide parents to keep bedside areas free of loud noises by showing them how to close bedside doors quietly and to limit adult conversation in close proximity to their infant. Encourage them to bring preterm infants nonnoise-producing items such as soft blankets and knitted hats or booties. Explain that musical toys should be used when the infant is older and more tolerant of noises.

Infants 26 to 27 Weeks Gestation

Infants at this age are unable to tolerate much stimulation. Instead, they need developmental supports that reduce stress and promote sleep. Encourage parents to look at their infant closely before beginning any interaction. When the infant is in quiet sleep, help parents understand the importance of sleep to the infant's well-being and reinforce that their infant's primary task is to sleep and grow.

Once the infant begins to move or shows signs of waking, assist parents to begin their interactions by first speaking softly to their infant (see Figure 6–8). When infants open their eyes in response to a vocalization, guide parents to stop talking and to keep their face close

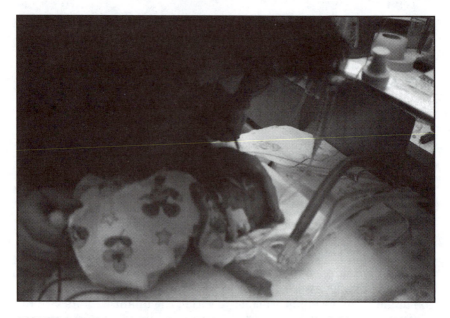

FIGURE 6–8. Parent interaction. (Photograph courtesy of Children's Hospital of Buffalo Department of Medical Photography.)

to their infant's face for several seconds. But do not stay there too long because at this age infants can tolerate only short periods of visual stimulation. Help parents recognize time-out signals such as turning away or closing eyes (Shapiro, 1992).

Infants 28 to 30 Weeks Gestation

If the infant is in an isolette, show parents how to shield the top portion of the isolette with a blanket to reduce any direct overhead lighting. Encourage parents to first look closely at their infant, determine the infant's state, and whether an intervention is appropriate. If in a quiet state, efforts should be made to maintain sleep. If the infant is in a quiet alert state, this is an optimal time to initiate interaction. Encourage parents to stay within their infant's visual field when speaking. In this way the infant will begin to associate the sound of the parent's voice with the parent's face.

If the infant can be held, demonstrate swaddling the infant's arms at midline and the infant's hands close to his or her face. Fold one edge of the infant's blanket over the infant's forehead to act as a shield against the nursery lighting. Infants will often open their eyes if nursery lighting is blocked.

Guide parents to begin by just holding their infant quietly. Then they should talk to their infant and watch the infant's cues. If the infant tolerates both holding and vocalization, guide parents to add other stimuli such as touching and rocking. Again, be certain they watch their infant's reaction to each added stimuli. Help parents recognize that gaze aversion, yawning, sleep, lethargy, or a glazed stare may be time-out cues.

Infants 31 to 32 Weeks Gestation

At this gestational age quiet alert states are increasingly frequent periods. Encourage parents to talk to their infant for longer periods during these times. Musical toys or tape recordings of the parents' voices are appropriate now. Guide parents to continue watching their infant's reaction especially to new types of stimulation.

Have parents hold their infant in a vertical position and move the infant from side to side horizontally. This motion will stimulate the infant to open its eyes. Help parents understand that an infant of this gestational age is beginning to focus and track items in its visual field now and will benefit from seeing them. Place toys within the infant's visual field, a distance of 8 to 10 inches. If possible change the toys within the infant's visual field (see Figure 6–9).

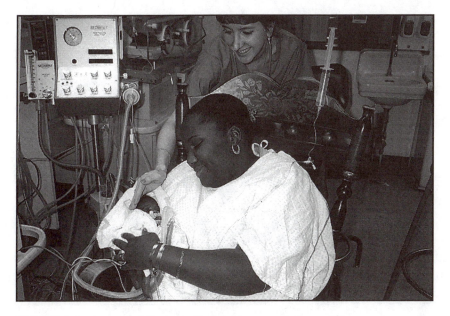

FIGURE 6–9. Parent interaction with infant on a ventilator. (Photograph courtesy of Children's Hospital of Buffalo Department of Medical Photography.)

Again, it is important to match interventions to each infant. If the infant is a stable growing premature baby, caregivers may feel very comfortable using interventions described in this chapter. However, if a premature infant is admitted to the NICU with acute medical needs, many of the interventions described would be inappropriate.

Infants 33 to 35 Weeks Gestation

Infants should visually follow an object at this gestational age. Encourage parents to bring in a hanging mobile. Show parents how to position the mobile within infant's visual field, but away from direct lighting.

At this gestational age infants begin to show visual preferences. Encourage parents to discover their infant's visual preferences for the bedside toys. Suggest that parents try visual toys consisting of contrasting patterns and human faces.

Show parents how to cover the upper edge of a bassinet with a blanket to help protect the infant from overhead lighting during sleep time (see Figure 6–10).

Let parents know that any interaction may overwhelm their infant and that they can comfort their infant. First they need to under-

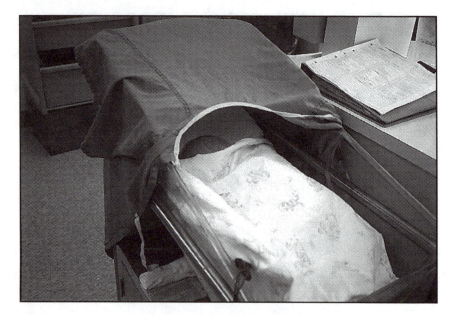

FIGURE 6–10. Infant in covered bassinet. (Photograph courtesy of Children's Hospital of Buffalo Department of Medical Photography.)

stand what their infant's signals mean. When they see time-out cues, they should either stop the interaction and quietly hold their infant or offer a rest period free of interaction.

Infants 36 to 38 Weeks Gestation

Explain to parents that their infant at this gestational age will be most alert just after feeding or between feedings. Encourage parents to be aware of these times and prepare for interactions when their infant is in an alert state.

These infants will be able to follow an item in all directions provided the item is moving within the infant's visual field. Show the parents this skill by having them move from side to side after their infant has focused visually on them. Encourage parents to leave their infant's favorite toys within the infant's visual field, approximately 8 to 10 inches from the infant. Guide them to periodically change the items within the infant's visual field. Encourage parents to use pictures with face-like patterns or photographs of the faces of family members.

Encourage parents to change positions while speaking to their infant. This change of position provides the infant with sounds from many directions. For an alert infant who can tolerate longer periods of stimulation, have parents repeat the infant's name or sing a song several times. Such repetition provides the infant with audibly predictable stimuli.

■ RECOMMENDATIONS FOR NICU CAREGIVERS

The following suggestions will help NICU caregivers protect and nurture the premature infants in their care. Some of the suggestions deal with caregiver actions; others address NICU practice and policies. For convenience, the suggestions are arranged under three different but related goals.

Goal 1: Limit constant and excessive handling of infants in the NICU.

Suggestions:

- ■ Use proper handling and positioning techniques.
- ■ Begin the infant's care by assessing the infant's state. If the infant is in a quiet sleep state, delay care until later if possible.
- ■ Touch the infant slowly and gently.
- ■ Turn infants using quarter turn movements. Wait between quarter turns for the infant to recover.
- ■ Help infants self-regulate by positioning their arms at midline with hands close to mouth.

- Be aware of the infant's cues and plan interventions accordingly.

Goal 2: Eliminate constant, excessively bright lighting in the NICU.
Suggestions:

- Use knitted caps that cover the head and eyes. Some nurseries have local church groups that knit these caps for the infants. When the infant is discharged home, the little cap also goes home too for the infant's baby book.
- Use stockinette like a headband. Place it over the infant's head, covering the eyes and ears.
- If the infant is under a plastic heat shield, use a cloth diaper to cover the upper portion of the heat shield and help block out light.
- Drape blankets over isolettes and bassinets to block out overhead lighting. Some nurseries use handmade covers for the isolette. These covers can then be used as baby blankets when the infant goes home.
- Institute a quiet time within the nursery when all lights are dimmed.

Goal 3: Diminish the constant, excessively loud noise in the NICU.
Suggestions:

- Be alert to increases in the noise level of the unit.
- Cover ears of infants who are acutely ill with stockinette padded with cotton.
- Decrease extraneous noise such as telephones, radios, loud conversation, and unchecked monitor alarms.
- Refrain from yelling messages across the unit or holding conversations over an infant.
- Close equipment doors and trash can lids quietly; pad trash can lids to decrease noise.
- Closely watch for infant's reaction to musical toys. If the infant becomes hyperactive or hypotonic, remove the musical stimuli.

■ SUMMARY

Developmental interventions are interventions that promote stability by protecting or stimulating premature infants. Developmental interventions do not need to be complex. They can be as easy as turning an infant slowly and gently while flexing its arms and legs. Several basic steps needed to provide appropriate interventions for each specific infant.

The first step is to assess the infant's capabilities and states. Look at the infant. Watch the infant. Through assessment, NICU caregivers can decide what, if any, interventions are appropriate. If the infant is in a quiet sleep, hands on interventions are not appropriate. Decreasing light and noise are appropriate. They will help the infant's slumber continue uninterrupted.

Understand the developmental skills of premature infants. Each infant has developmental needs based on physical condition and gestational age. The basic developmental skills of each gestational age group are available in journals and texts. Another way to understand the developmental needs of preterm infants is by caring for them. Parents often learn what is developmentally appropriate for their infant by carefully watching their infant's reaction to various stimuli.

Caregivers can incorporate developmental interventions as a part of their routine daily care in the intensive care nursery. Swaddling an infant after an invasive procedure such as a heelstick or controlling the lighting over an infant by covering the isolette are developmental interventions.

Finally, there needs to be a sensitive network of communication among all the infant's caregivers, be they health care professionals or family members. Communication among caregivers is critical for revising and tailoring developmental interventions for each infant. It is communication among all an infant's caregivers that results in developmental interventions being infant specific and infant appropriate.

Providing developmentally appropriate interventions is a relatively straightforward process:

■ carefully observe infants
■ gather information about the appropriate developmental interventions for each specific gestational age group
■ actively incorporate developmental interventions into daily infant care
■ talk to parents and to NICU health professionals about the responses you see in the infant.

> *Infants are always the only future the*
> *human race has...teach them well.*
> Anonymous

■ REFERENCES

Affonso, D. D., Hurst, I., Mayberry, L. J., Haller, L., Yost, K. & Lynch, M. E. (1992). Stressors reported by mothers of hospitalized premature infants. *Neonatal Network, 11*(6), 63–70

Als, H. (1982). Toward a synactive theory of development: Promise for the assessment and support of infant individuality. *Infant Mental Health Journal, 3*(4), 229–243.

Als, H. (1986). A synactive model of neonatal behavioral organization: Framework for assessment of neurobehavioral development in the premature infant and for the support of infants and parents in the neonatal intensive care environment. *Physical and Occupational Therapy in Pediatrics, 6*, 3–53.

Als, H., Lawhon,. G., Duffy, F., McAnulty, G. B., Gibes-Grossman, R., & Blickman, J. G. (1994). Individualized developmental care for the very low-birthweight preterm infant: Medical and neurofunctional effects. *Journal of the American Medical Association, 272*(11), 853–858.

Anderson, J. (1986). Sensory intervention with the preterm infant in the neonatal intensive care unit. *American Journal of Occupational Therapy, 40*(1), 19–26.

Aumann, G. M-E., (1988). New chances, new choices: Problems with perinatal technology. *Journal of Perinatal and Neonatal Nursing, 1*(3), 1–9.

Avery, M. E., & Taeusch, H. W. (Eds.). (1984). *Schaffer's diseases of the newborn*. Philadelphia: W. B. Saunders.

Beachy, P., & Deacon, J. (Eds.). (1993). *Core curriculum for neonatal intensive care nursing*. Philadelphia: W. B. Saunders.

Belsky, J. (1984). The determinants of parenting: A process model. *Child Development, 55*, 83–96.

Brazleton, T. B., (1975). Anticipatory guidance. *Pediatric Clinics of North America, 22*(33), 533–544.

Burns, K., Cunningham, N., White-Traut, R., Silvestri, J., & Nelson, M. N. (1994). Infant stimulation: Modification of an intervention based on psysiologic and behavioral cues. *Journal of Obstetric, Gynecologic and Neonatal Nursing, 23*(7), 581–590.

Creger, P. J. (1993). Developmental support in the NICU. In P. Beachy & J. Deacon (Eds.), *Core curriculum for neonatal intensive care nursing* (pp. 426–442). Philadelphia: W. B. Saunders.

Creger, P. J., & Browne, J. V. (Eds.). (1989). *Developmental interventions for preterm and high-risk infants*. Tucson, AZ: Therapy Skill Builders.

Cusson, R. M., & Lee, A. L. (1993). Parental interventions and the development of the preterm infant. *Journal of Obstetric, Gynecologic and Neonatal Nursing, 23*(1), 60–68.

DeCasper, A. J., & Fifer, W. P. (1983). Of human bonding: Newborns prefer their mother's voices. *Science, 208*, 1175.

Dunham, C., Myers, F., Barnden, N., McDougall, Al, Kelly, T. L., & Aria, B (1991). *Mamatoto*. New York: Viking Penquin.

Field, T. (1990). *Infancy*. Cambridge: Harvard University Press.

Freiberg, K. (1992). *Human development: A life-span approach*. Boston: Jones and Bartlett.

Gardner, S. L., Garland, K. R., Merenstein, S. L., & Merenstein, G. B. (1989). The neonate and the environment: Impact on development. In G. B. Merenstein & S. L. Gardner (Eds.), *Handbook of neonatal intensive care* (pp. 628–675). St. Louis: C. V. Mosby.

Heriza, C. B., & Sweeney, J. K. (1990). Effects of NICU intervention on preterm infants: Part I: Implications for neonatal practice. *Infants and Young Children, 2*(3), 31–47.

Kenner, C., & Lott, J. W. (1990). Parent transition after discharge from the NICU. *Neonatal Network, 9*(2), 31–37.

Langman, J. (1991). In T. W. Sadler, (Ed.), *Langman's medical embryology* (6th edition). Baltimore: Williams & Wilkins.

Lyons, J. (1985). *Playing god in the nursery*. New York: W. W. Norton.

Mann, N. P., Haddow, R., Stokes, L., Goodley, S., & Rutter, N. (1986). Effect of night and day on preterm infants in a newborn nursery: Randomised trial. *British Medical Journal, 293*, 1265–1267.

McMillen, C., Kok, J. S., Adamson, T. M., Deayton, J. M., & Nowak, R. (1991). Development of circadian sleep-wake rhythms in preterm and full-term infants. *Pediatric Research, 29*(4), 381–384.

Medoff-Cooper, B. (1988). The effects of handling on premature infants with bronchopulmonary dysplasia. *Image: Journal of Nursing Scholarship, 20*(3), 132–134.

Miles, M. S. (1989). Parents of critically ill premature infants, sources of stress. *Critical Care Nursing Quarterly, 12*(3), 69–74.

Peters, K. L. (1992). Does routine nursing care complicate the physiologic status of the premature neonate with respiratory distress syndrome? *Journal of Perinatal and Neonatal Nursing, 20*(3), 132–134.

Pridham, K. F. (1993). Anticipatory guidance of parents of new infants: Potential contribution of the internal working model. *Image, 25*(1), 49–56.

Rosenberg, C. E. (1987). *The case of strangers: The rise of America's hospital system*. New York: Basic Books.

Shapiro, C. (1992). Opthalmologic disorders. In P. Beachy & J. Deacon (Eds.), *Core curriculum for neonatal intensive care nursing* (pp. 485–450). Philadelphia: W. B. Saunders.

Thoman, E. B., Ingersall, E. W., & Acebo, C. (1991). Premature infants seek rhythmic stimulation, and the experience facilitates neurobehavioral development. *Developmental and Behavioral Pediatrics, 12*(1), 11–18.

VandenBerg, K. (1985). Revising the traditional model: An individualized approach to developmental interventions in the intensive care nursery. *Neonatal Network, 3*, 32–38.

Velasco-Whetsell, M., Evans, J., & Wang, M. (1992). Do postsuctioning transcutaneous PO_2 values change when a neonate's movements are restrained? *Journal of Perinatology, 7*(4), 333–337.

White-Traut, R. C., Nelson, M. N., Burns, K., & Cunningham, N. (1994). Environmental influences on the developing premature infant: Theoretical issues and applications to practice. *Journal of Obstetrics, Gynecologic, and Neonatal Nursing, 23*, 393–401.

Witt, C. L. (1993). Neonatal dermatology. In P. Beachy & J. Deacon (Eds.), *Core curriculum for neonatal intensive care nursing* (pp. 471–474). Philadelphia: W. B. Saunders.

Yecco, G. S. (1993). Neuro behavioral development and developmental support of premature infants. *Journal of Perinatal and Neonatal Nursing,* 7(1), 56–85.

Yoos, L. (1989). Applying research in practice: Parenting the premature infant. *Applied Nursing Research, 2*(1), 30–34.

■ CHAPTER 7

Parent-Preterm Infant Interactions

Accidents will happen in the
best regulated families.
Charles DIckens

■ INTRODUCTION

It is both delightful and wonderful to see babies and their parents smiling, exchanging glances, and enjoying one another. Our delight grows out of the evident joy in such exchanges. Our wonder centers on the importance of the budding relationships.

It is no exaggeration to argue that the early relationship between parents and their infant is the cornerstone of an infant's development. Early interactions establish trust and security. They enable infants to develop the healthy emotional ties so important to the attachment process.

Premature infants and their families have very different beginnings. Parents are rarely prepared for their first view of their tiny baby hooked up to monitors. Instead of beginning interactions with their baby, parents' focus may be on whether the baby will live. Their initial communications will be with medical staff rather than their baby.

> I gave birth to Michael in a small suburban hospital. He was two months early so he was rushed to a larger unit. My husband saw him first. It was three days before I saw him. I was stunned to see how tiny he was.
>
> Our baby was born nine weeks premature. She had a lot of serious medical problems. It was very hard on us because we didn't know whether she would live. She did not look or act like the baby we had expected. Gradually we got acquainted. It was a slow process and the nurses were there to help us out.

Research on parent-preterm interaction and attachment in the NICU has shown that parents feel alienated and often have initial difficulty forming attachments with their infants (Freund, 1988; Parker, Zahr, Cole, & Brecht, 1992). Other investigators have looked more closely at the individual experiences and priorities of families and their needs while they are in the NICU and after discharge (Bass, 1991; McHaffie, 1992; Perlman et al., 1991). Family interventions are being implemented to support family involvement with their hospitalized infants and in their transition from hospital to home (Gennaro, Brooten, & Bakewell-Sachs, 1991; Rushton, 1990).

In this chapter, we will focus on the impact of prematurity on parent-infant interactions. First, we will examine the social interactional patterns typical of full-term infants, then look at factors that affect parent-infant interactions in the NICU. Other interactions in the NICU and the impact of problematic interaction patterns will be described. Finally, we will suggest interventions for facilitating positive preterm infant-parent interactions in the intensive care nursery.

■ FORMING ATTACHMENTS: THE FULL-TERM INFANT

Human newborns are remarkably well organized for developing an affectional bond with their caregivers. The first steps in the complex process of attachment begin within hours after birth. Newborn senses and behaviors are ready to begin an interactive process with their caregivers that involves mutual synchrony and regulation (Coll & Meyer,1993). With enough practice and exposure, a lasting attachment is formed between parent and infant (see Figure 7–1).

Newborns' Capacity for Attachment

Newborns seem to be equipped to respond to special features of the adults around them. They can distinguish their own mothers' voices from those of other adult females (DeCasper & Fifer, 1980). According to Macfarlane (1975), infants older than 6 days turn their head more often in the direction of a pad saturated with their mother's breast milk than to a pad with the breast milk of a strange woman. Newborns will look at their caregiver's face and then move their bodies toward the caregiver (Maurer & Maurer, 1988). Other investigations found that as early as 1 month infants distinguish speech from nonspeech sounds (Eimas, Siqueland, Jusczyk, & Vigorito, 1971). Infants as young as 12 days old are able to imitate adults' facial gestures such as tongue protrusion and mouth opening (Meltzoff & Moore, 1977, 1989).

Neonatal cries are effective early communication signals to parents. Infants signal their caregivers using a variety of cries (Zeskind

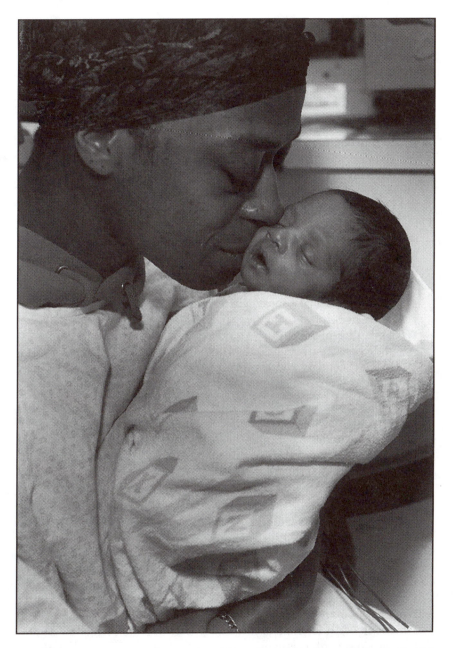

FIGURE 7–1. A preterm infant receives his mother's kiss. (Photograph courtesy of Children's Hospital of Buffalo Department of Medical Photography.)

& Lester, 1978, 1981). Adults can distinguish differences in the cries whether they are cries of pain or general distress. The cries of infants evoke responses from adults such as talking, touching, rocking, or holding the infants (Gustafson & Harris, 1990). The caregivers' responses are essential to the attachment process.

Many newborn behaviors help them establish an affectional bond with their caregivers. Some of these behaviors include:

- Self-arousing to an alert state; this allows infants to attend to interesting events in their environment.
- Actively fixating on attractive visual stimuli and quieting while watching visually interesting moving objects.
- Demonstrating preference for certain sounds or sights by shutting eyes or covering face.
- Quieting from a crying state to listen to a soft human voice.
- Using cries to communicate needs.
- Using signaling responses to elicit contingent responses from caregivers.
- Moving the body in synchrony with the words and sounds made by adults.
- Engaging in mutual turntaking with caregivers. For example, the caregiver looks at the baby and vocalizes, the baby quiets, looks at the caregiver, and then moves her body in response to the caregiver's sounds.

Such behaviors tell us that adults and newborn infants are ready to interact with one another. Very early in an infant's life, caregivers adapt their behaviors to match those of the infant. This process, often referred to as the "dance between infant and caregiver," results in attachment (Klaus & Robertson, 1982).

As they mature, infants become more skilled at initiating and terminating their interactions with caregivers. In fact, they soon control approximately 90% of the interactions. Their early messages to caregivers are simple and direct, usually involving movements, sounds, or visual gazing. With increasing maturity, infants send more complex signals involving combinations of visual, auditory, and movement stimuli (Cohn & Elmore, 1988). Caregivers in turn respond and a reciprocal "dance" is firmly established between the two partners (Thoman & Browder,1987). The dance is synchronous and harmonious, with feelings of mutuality that are the core of successful caregiver-infant interactions.

Many important behaviors and interaction patterns contribute to establishing a relationship between developing infants and their caregivers (Fogel & Thelen, 1987). Included are the following:

Mutual gaze. Shortly after birth, infants gaze into the eyes of their caregivers who in turn gaze back. This behavior is known as "mutual gaze" and is a first step in attachment (Stern, 1982). As infants develop, the gaze period lengthens and involves verbal and motor play between caregivers and infant.

Smiling. Smiling can elicit adult-infant interactions. Newborn smiles are termed "endogenous" and occur spontaneously, but caregivers often interpret the smiles to be directed at them. By the third month of life, smiling becomes more social and specifically directed toward caregivers (Emde, Gaensbauer, & Harmon, 1976).

Imitation. When caregivers imitate their infant's body movements, sounds, and facial expressions, they help sustain their baby's attention (Metzoff & Moore, 1989). Such imitation also provides predictability. Adult imitation establishes early rhythmic interactions which over time become more "gamelike" between infant and caregiver. As infants develop, they begin to imitate the caregiver's actions and anticipate what the caregiver is about to do.

Contingency and responsivity. Infants learn to adjust their responses to the feedback they receive from their caregivers. Their contingent responses become more and more complex as they mature. These responses are a critical part of the process by which infants learn they can affect their environment.

Synchrony. Newborns move their bodies in synchrony with adult speech (Condon & Sander, 1974). As infants develop, the synchrony between infant and caregiver becomes more obvious in their games, communication and social interactions. Synchronous behaviors between infants and caregivers involve physical movements, facial gestures, and use of sounds and words.

Games. Caregivers engage their infants in simple games to elicit social responses and thereby involve infants in contingent learning. They may handle their infant in a playful way or play "peek-a-boo." The games become more varied and complex as infants develop. During their games, the parent-infant partners imitate each other and provide feedback. Their message to each other is, "You're special to me."

Positive Outcomes of Reciprocal Interactions

Engaging in and completing a successful attachment process results in a strong reciprocal bond that is the cornerstone for subsequent developmental outcomes. Positive outcomes for both infants and caregivers are involved (Fogel, 1991). The following are positive outcomes:

■ Infants develop autonomy and a sense of self-emergence.

■ Infants learn about themselves and their environment.

- Infants learn ways to control their environment.
- Infants' cognitive development is promoted.
- Both infants and caregivers acquire feelings of competence.
- Interactions serve as a basis for later communication.
- Infants and caregivers learn to adapt to one another and to continually modify their interactions.
- An ongoing relationship between infants and caregivers develops and grows.
- The infants have a base for generalizing appropriate interactions with others.
- A rewarding experience occurs for both infants and caregivers.

■ FACTORS THAT JEOPARDIZE PARENT-PRETERM INFANT INTERACTIONS

NICU infants and their caregivers do not always experience the positive results of a successful attachment process. For some, a rewarding reciprocal infant-caregiver relationship is firmly established in the NICU; but for others, the relationship is not reciprocal. Instead a frustrating interactive experience occurs between caregiver and infant. Reasons for this and ways to assist caregivers and infants in developing supportive interactions will be addressed in the remainder of the chapter.

Preterm-parent interactions are influenced by a complex array of factors that involve the infant, the family and the NICU environment. There are many factors that jeopardize the development of supportive interaction patterns between preterm infants and their parents (Field, 1979; Minde, 1993). For example, infants are often not as capable of responding to the demands of social interaction. Their parents' social behavior may be qualitatively different within the context of the NICU.

For preterm infants in the NICU, the development of normal interactional processes so essential to attachment may be altered by many factors including the NICU milieu, the infant's vulnerability, and the parents' perceptions of their infant. While preterm infants develop affectional ties with caregivers using the same mechanisms as full-term infants, the attachment process may be much slower and difficult to identify because of their immaturity, medical state and unresponsiveness. The behavioral characteristics of preterm infants may affect the parent-infant interactional dyad. The reciprocal and synchronous behaviors that characterize healthy full-term infant and parent interactions may be compromised in the social beginnings of premature infants and their parents. The desired match between caregiver and infant may not occur, and this can have long-term deleterious consequences for the infant's well-being and subsequent interactions.

Interactions may be influenced by the infant's capabilities and medical condition. The NICU environment may affect an infant's temperament and functioning as an effective social partner. Parents' social behaviors are also affected by the NICU experience. They must try to initiate social beginnings within the context of bright lights, noise, and lack of privacy, and the stress associated with a premature birth can alter parents' interactions with their infants. Parents may view their premature infant as less social, less competent, and less likeable than a full-term infant (Stern & Karraker, 1990). This may be exaggerated among parents and infants from low socioeconomic conditions where a number of cumulative risk factors have been identified.

Premature Infants

Characteristics of premature infants can alter the social dynamics between them and parents. In fact, early social encounters of premature infants and their caregivers can differ dramatically (Lester, Hoffman, & Brazelton, 1985). Most premature infants are unable to interact actively with their caregivers. In part this is due to the characteristics and capabilities premature infants bring to the social encounters. Often premature infants in the intensive care nursery are fragile and physically unable to give clear attachment signals. Sometimes they give no signals at all. Very low birthweight infants frequently experience a variety of medical problems that place them at medical risk, for example, apnea, bradycardia, hypoxia, and respiratory distress syndrome. Their precarious medical state results in disorganized behavioral responses or an inability to stabilize their social interactions. Social encounters may be nonexistent or very different from their full-term counterparts.

Being born too soon means that premature babies' central nervous system may be considerably less developed than the nervous system of term babies. Premature infants, for example, have greater difficulty regulating autonomic responses and states (Prechtl, Fargel, Weinmann, & Bakker, 1979). They have been found to cry less and with less vigor than full-term infants (Divitto & Goldberg, 1979). Compared to full-term newborns, premature infants with an immature nervous system may not be predisposed to respond to interaction stimuli such as a father's or mother's touch (Eckerman & Oehler, 1992). When they do respond, their behavioral cues may be markedly different than the behavioral cues of full-term infants. Their cues to caregivers may be weaker, more difficult to read, or be primarily avoidance cues such as gaze aversion or crying.

Because of preterm infants' neurological immaturity their behaviors may be organizationally different from the behaviors of full-term infants. Preterm infants are less responsive, and they are easily taxed by environmental stimulation. Although they are difficult to arouse, once this happens they become overaroused and hypersensitive to environmental input (Aylward, 1982). Compared to full-term infants, preterm infants have weaker and fewer cries, less well-developed rooting and sucking responses, and poorer hand to mouth maneuvers in feeding interactions (Brown & Bakeman, 1979). Adaptation to sights and sounds so characteristic of healthy full-term infants is not evident in sick or very low birthweight infants.

Even older, more intact premature infants show immature responses and disorganized social orientation patterns. Rose (1983) found that older premature infants born close to full-term show less behavioral responsiveness to tactile stimulation, longer active sleep periods, and a low correlation between change in heart rate and behavioral activation. Older premature infants born close to 40 weeks have been described as less alert and responsive, with poor motor and state modulation (Alfasi et al., 1985; Minde, Perrotta, & Marton, 1985).

At discharge, premature infants have been shown to do more poorly than full-term infants on attention and interaction items from the Brazelton Neonatal Behavioral Assessment Scale (Brazelton, 1973; Lester, Emory, Hoffman, & Eitzman, 1976). McGehee and Eckerman (1983) assessed the behavioral responses to social stimulation of very low birthweight premature infants and full-term infants at the time of hospital discharge. Infants were exposed to tactile, visual, auditory, and combined auditory and tactile social stimulation. Preterm infants, although responsive to the stimuli, had different patterns of response organization. Preterm infants exhibited frequent shifts in state, more erratic jerky movements, and gasps and grunts. These responses are thought to present "unreadable" social cues to the caregiver. Field (1979) found that older high-risk preterm infants engaged in more gaze aversion and were more fussy in face-to-face interactions with their mother.

A key component in any parent-infant interaction is the signaling behavior of each member of the dyad. If they are to enable parents to correctly read, interpret, and respond appropriately to their signals, an infant's behaviors and cries must be clear. For premature infants, particularly very young premature ones, communication cues are unclear at best. Mixed or confusing signals of premature infants make it difficult for caregivers to respond appropriately.

Parents

Parents of preterm infants differ, too. They have unique experiences that can alter the early social encounters with their infant. Unlike parents of full-term infants, they may feel unprepared for the premature delivery. The unanticipated premature infant's arrival sets in motion a new series of unexpected events and crises. Usually parents are separated from their baby resulting in feelings of isolation (McCluskey-Fawcett, O'Brien, Robinson, & Asay, 1992). Parents who must commute long distances may visit their infants more infrequently, consequently making it more difficult to establish a bond with their infant. Family members and friends who ordinarily would congratulate the new parents, may not know what to say or do in the event of a premature birth.

Parents may not be able to cope with the serious medical condition of their infant and with the crisis and ambiguity of the infant's precarious state. An early birth is often accompanied by intense feelings of anxiety, guilt, and grief. Parents may feel overwhelmed by a rollercoaster of emotions as their baby's condition worsens or improves. Some parents will distance themselves emotionally from their baby, fearing the baby might die.

Parents who expected a rosy-cheeked, healthy baby may be distressed by their first view of their infant in the NICU. The baby may be tiny and scrawny with few of the expected "normal" baby features. The baby's skin may be wrinkled, giving an old appearance. The baby may not open her eyes at all or her eyes may be covered by eye coverings. It may even be difficult to see the baby because of the many tubes and monitor leads attached to her body.

At the same time, parents must attempt to cope with the overwhelming medical technology of the NICU coupled with the high noise level, 24-hour lighting, and infant isolation. Unlike the home environment, the NICU is filled with activity and many people. There is little privacy for parents to interact or be alone with their baby. Sick babies will be surrounded by monitors and have tubes coming from various parts of their body, making them inaccessible for viewing or touching. Parents are often hesitant to initiate interactions or routine care such as a diaper change even when their baby is stable because they feel less competent than the NICU staff. Such conditions make it easy to understand why being a high-risk infant in an intensive care nursery increases the likelihood that healthy parent-infant interactions may be jeopardized.

Parents' individual characteristics may also affect psychosocial interactions with their infant. Parents of premature infants have been shown to experience negative emotions and heightened stress (Culp, Applebaum, Osofsky, & Levy, 1988). The difficult life events and increased stress associated with parenting a premature infant may elicit depression. Depressed mothers have been shown to be detached and withdrawn in their interactions with their infants (Cohn, Matias, Tronick, Lyons-Ruth, & Connell, 1986). Another study found that infants at risk for developmental problems because of intraventricular hemorrhage (IVH) may be at further developmental risk as a result of mothers' depressive responsiveness to them (Wilfong, Saylor, & Elksnin, 1991).

Parents' perceptions of what premature babies are like may also influence subsequent interactions with their own premature infant. Their perceptions are influenced by their expectations of parenthood, family history, education, and marital relationships. Despite the variety of backgrounds and experiences parents bring to the NICU, studies have shown that they have preconceived ideas about premature babies. These perceptions are often negatively biased toward premature infants.

Stern and Hildebrandt (1984) asked mothers to interact with healthy full-term babies who were labeled as either full term or premature. Mothers who believed they were interacting with premature infants touched them less and gave them more immature toys than did the mothers who believed they were interacting with "full-term" babies. "Premature" infants were also rated as less active, more fragile, and less cute than the "full-term" infants (Stern & Hildebrant, 1986; Stern & Karraker, 1990).

Prematurity prejudice was found in another study in which mothers of premature infants viewed videotapes of full-term infants who had been labeled either full term or premature (Stern & Karraker, 1988). The "premature" infants were perceived as weaker, smaller, slower, and more passive that the "full-term" infants. Despite the fact that the babies on video appeared healthy and active, mothers of preterm infants apparently had biased expectations of premature infants' looks and behaviors. Similar findings of adult prematurity prejudice was found by Miller and Ottinger (1988) and by Epps (1993) with nurses in neonatal intensive care units.

Parents' biased perceptions of premature infants can persist even after discharge from the NICU. Washington, Minde, and Goldberg (1986) asked mothers of 3- and 6-month premature infants to rate their infants' temperaments using the Infant Temperament Questionnaire (Carey & McDivitt, 1978). Thomas and Chess (1977) described temperament as a behavioral style consisting of nine temperament traits: initial approach-withdrawal, adaptability, activity, biologic rhythmicity, mood quality, persistence, distractibility, intensity of reaction, and sensory threshold. Full-term babies rated, using the Infant Temperament Questionnaire, were found to fall in three temperament categories: easy, slow-to-warm up, and difficult.

Parents of premature infants rated their babies as having a more difficult temperament compared to full-term infants (Washington et al., 1986). In a comparison study of mother's temperament ratings of their premature infants at 6 months of age, Spungen and Farran (1986) found that mothers rated high-risk preterm infants as more difficult than low-risk preterm infants. The length of the infants' hospitalization and severity of medical involvement accounted for the mothers' perceptions of their infants after hospitalization.

NICU Environment

The NICU environment affects both parents and infants. Premature infants spend their early life in an environment that differs greatly from the home environment of full-term infants (Hayes & Ensher, 1994). Preterm infants in the NICU are exposed to more adult speech and infant cries than are full-term infants at home. They experience more noncontingent social speech and higher levels of noise and light that are associated with the technology of the intensive care nursery. Speech sounds are distorted for infants in incubators.

Parents may find the bright lights, loud noise, and lack of privacy deter interactions with their infant in the NICU. NICUs with limited visiting hours may have an additional negative effect on parents' involvement with their infant. Interaction patterns of parents in NICUs with limited visiting hours with those in NICUs with unlimited visiting hours. Thirteen percent of the parents in the limited visiting situation did not interact with their infants when they were in an incubator, compared to only 2.2% of the parents in the unlimited visiting NICU (Paludetto, Dell'Antonio, DeCurtis, DeVito, & DiVito, 1984).

NICU staff may also present barriers to parents' involvement and subsequent interaction with their infant. NICU staff may be unwilling to allow parents to participate in their infant's care. Parental decision making and involvement may be viewed negatively by staff who feel parents will usurp their role (Griffin, 1990). In a recent study, parents who reported the most positive experiences in the intensive care nursery were those who NICU staff viewed as interested and capable of caring for their infants (McCluskey-Fawcett et al., 1992).

■ PARENT-INFANT INTERACTIONS IN THE NICU

Concern for the psychosocial outcomes of high-risk infants in the nursery has lagged behind the NICU's increasingly sophisticated lifesaving practices and activities. Recently, however, increasing attention has been given to the social interactional patterns of premature infants and parents in the NICU as well as interventions that promote supportive interventions. Because these infants have been prematurely thrust into the extrauterine world, they are often ill equipped to meet the challenges of social interactions (DiVitto & Goldberg, 1979). Early social communication, which is especially important for parents of newborns, may be missing for parents of premature infants.

A premature birth can alter parent-infant interactions (Minde, Whitelaw, Brown, & Fitzhardinge, 1983). Observational studies of parent-preterm infant interaction patterns have identified interactional disturbances that are predictive of developmental difficulties later in infancy (Field, 1982).

Recent studies have shown that while interactive difficulties are often evident during early hospitalization of preterm infants, it is not a certainty that families and their infants will have long-term interactional problems. The length and severity of post-preterm interactional problems depends on early intervention aimed at ameliorating such difficulties (Brooks-Gunn, Liaw, & Klebanov, 1992; Lee, Penner, & Cox, 1991). Further, social interactions between parents and their high-risk infants may be qualitatively different from the interactions between parents and full-term infants. Parents who attempt to visually engage their preterm infant may experience gaze aversion rather than a mutual gaze. A comparison of the interaction patterns of full-term and preterm infants with their parents revealed that the interaction of preterm infants and their mothers were less synchronous and coordinated than those of full-term infants (Lester et al., 1985). Goldson (1992) suggested that parents' sense of competence may be compromised by their child's premature birth and the nature of the NICU environment, which makes it less likely they will engage their baby in interactions.

Because preterm infants provide fewer social cues to parents in the interactive process, parents must expend more energy to maintain a social exchange. Als (1979) documented preterm infants' low level of responsiveness to social stimuli and their parents' increased but futile efforts to sustain interaction. In 1978, Goldberg reviewed the existing literature on preterm-parent interaction. She concluded that mothers of premature infants worked harder at getting their infant's attention but were less successful than mothers of full-term infants.

In face-to-face interactions between preterm infants and their mothers, Field (1977) found mothers used more "intrusive" interactive behaviors such as overstimulation and control to elicit infant response. Other studies supported these findings. Mothers were more actively involved in feeding their preterm infants. They touched and talked to the infants in efforts to engage them socially. These were largely one-way interactions, with the mother acting alone and receiving little positive feedback or no feedback from her infant. As parents attempt to elicit responses from their preterm infants, the infants display more gaze aversion and turning away, which suggests that they are overstimulated (Goldberg, 1978).

While some interactional problems result from a mismatch of social exchanges between parent and infant, other problems are a function of the seriousness of the infant's medical condition and the parents' response to it. Infants with precarious medical complications at birth may present a serious crisis for parents expecting a healthy infant. The infant's medical condition can have a substantial impact on parents' perception of the infant. Their response may be to withdraw from the infant (Minde, 1992). Compared to parents of healthy full-term infants, parents of ill premature infants have been found to show less face-to-face contact, less smiling, less affectionate touching, and less talk in their interactions (Goldberg & DiVitto, 1983).

Parents' visiting patterns and their level of involvement with their infant also affect their interactions. Previous research on maternal visiting patterns showed that mothers who visited their infants less often, later had problems related to mothering (Farnaroff, Kennell, & Klaus, 1972). It was reported in another study that in the early periods after a premature infant's birth, interactions consisted principally of looking at the baby rather than active engagement. Mothers who visited over longer periods of time frequently were reported to become more actively involved with their infant (Minde et al., 1978).

Zeskind and Iacino (1984) assessed mothers' perceptions of their preterm infants when maternal visitation to the NICU was increased to regularly scheduled weekly visits. These mothers who had not been visiting regularly, were scheduled for weekly visits by their social workers. Mothers who increased their independent visitations had more positive perceptions of their infant's behavior. Infants in the visitation intervention group also had shorter hospital stays than infants in the control group. Moreover, the mothers' positive perceptions of the preterm infants in the visitation group continued after discharge. Rosenfield (1980) found that increased visitations by mothers of preterm infants were associated with more alert infants.

It appeared that contact even twice a week on a regular basis during infants' lengthy hospitalization facilitated the parent-infant bond.

The early research findings prompted a new look at family visitation policies in the NICU. Until the 1980s visitation policies largely excluded parents and other family members from the NICU (Plass, 1994). NICU health providers began to realize the negative impact of the separation of family and infant as well as the consequent stress on family members. In the mid 1980s, visitation policies began to change (Lewis et al., 1991). Parents were allowed to visit their infant for longer periods of time. Some NICUs implemented unlimited visiting hours. Sibling visitation became more widely accepted (Craft, Wyatt, & Sandell, 1985; Schwab, Tolbert, Bagnato, & Meisels, 1983). In addition, NICU staff began to encourage parents to become actively involved in the nonmedical aspects of their infant's care.

Most research on parent-infant interaction in the NICU has looked exclusively at the mother's relationship with her infant. The father's role with infants in the NICU was examined in several studies. Fathers often visit their baby in the NICU before mothers do. Marton, Minde, and Perrotta (1981), looked at fathers' visiting patterns and interactions with their infants. Fathers visited as often as mothers visited and they maintained equal levels of involvement with their infants over time. Moreover, this pattern of involvement continued after discharge from the hospital. Fathers of preterm infants were three times more likely than fathers of full-term infants to engage in infant caregiving such as feeding or bathing.

These findings on paternal parenting patterns were supported by other investigators. A more recent study examined fathering during the hospital stay, at discharge, at 8 months of age, and at 18 months of age. The frequency of fathers' hospital visits was found to be a significant predictor of the father's relationship with the infant and of the quality of the infant's development. When father-infant interaction patterns were more positive, infants were more likely to be discharged from the hospital earlier (Levy-Shiff, Hoffman, Mogilner, Levinger, & Mogilner, 1990).

Tinsley and Parke (1983) found no difference in the engagement levels of fathers and mothers of preterm infants in the hospital or after discharge. Further, they observed that both fathers and mothers smiled more and explored more with their baby when the other parent was present. They suggested that when both parents are present they support each other in developing positive exchanges with their preterm infant. Thurman and Korteland (1989) found that fathers interacted less with their infants in the NICU than did mothers. The parents communicated with their infant more often when alone than when together. Levy-Shiff, Sharir, and Mogilner (1989) looked at initial contacts between parents and their premature infant. Initially mothers engaged in more nurturant and interactive activities than did fathers, but by discharge, both parents engaged equally often in interactions such as talking and holding their infant.

While NICU preterm infants differ from full-term infants in their behavioral responsiveness to social stimuli and in their motor and state regulation, there is evidence that these behavioral differences can persist beyond the neonatal period. Garcia-Coll et al. (1987) reported that preterm infants with varying degrees of intraventricular hemorrhage showed less overall responses and activity up to 3 months corrected age. At 4 months, premature infants have been found to be more fretful and less attentive to interactive stimuli (Field, 1977). Crawford (1982) reported that premature infants of 6, 8, and 10 months vocalized less, played less and were more fussy than full-term infants of the same chronological age, but by 14 months the differences had disappeared. Several investigators have noted that during the first 6 months of life preterm infants have less verbal interaction, more negative affect, and give more distress signals (Macey, Harmon, & Easterbrooks, 1987). These persisting differences may put early parent-preterm infant interactions in jeopardy.

Interaction studies show that parent-preterm infant interactions differ significantly from full-term infants both during early infancy and during the infant's first year (Crnic, Ragozin, Greenberg, Robinson, & Basham, 1983). Mothers of very sick infants have been found to be less sensitive to their infant's cues and made less effective responses to infant distress at 4 and 8 months (Field, 1977; Jarvis, Myers, & Creasey, 1989).

Studies reviewed by Macey et al. (1987) show that the interactional differences of preterm infants and parents are still evident at 6 months and may last as long as 2 years. Despite the reported interaction disturbances, the attachment bond is relatively strong. The early interactions, however, may affect the quality of attachment.

■ SIGNS OF INTERACTIONAL DIFFICULTIES

In social interactions, fragile preterm infants are often unable to respond appropriately or even show signs of stress (Lawhon, 1986). Sometimes infants will attempt to respond to the caregiver, but the stimulation is simply too much and they escape it by looking away. Even brief interactions may tire a fragile infant to the point of overarousal. Developmental interventions must then assist the infant to self-regulate to a quiet state. Very small infants are usually not capable of sustaining any interactions because their energies are being expended for survival. Older, more stable infants may begin an interaction but are sometimes unable to sustain it.

Parents often lack confidence in interacting with their premature infant. They may not recognize the infant's interaction signals. Regardless of an infant's age, it is important to read the signs of stress. These signals tell caregivers to back off from interacting and to provide an environment that nurtures rather than taxes the infant's resources. Parents may interpret an infant's stress signs as rejection signals and think they are not doing enough to engage the infant to interact with them, when in fact the infant needs time out from any social interactions. Given these conditions, it is not surprising that interaction problems may occur.

Signs that interactions between parents and preterm infants are mismatched are:

Infant

- Gaze aversion
- Hyperarousal, unable to maintain control
- Disorganized responses
- Squirming away from adult voice or touch
- Being unresponsive to adult face or voice
- Eyes bulging, hyperalert look
- Expressions of discontent with the interaction (such as grimacing or covering the eyes or ears)
- Signs of physiological overload (such as color change or breathing problems)
- Fretting and fussiness
- Arms and legs in extension
- Back and head arching
- Going limp

Parent

- Does not notice the infant's behavioral and physiological cues that signal readiness to interact or to stop interacting.
- Misinterprets the infant's behavioral and physiological cues.
- Stimulates the infant excessively with too much movement or noise.
- Stimulates the infant inappropriately (for example, shakes an infant who is in a deep sleep state).
- Is passive (stands away from the infant and does not interact at all when the infant is alert and shows signs of wanting to interact).

■ Is hesitant (starts stimulation and then stops, even though the infant is alert and responding).

■ PROMOTING POSITIVE PARENT-PRETERM INFANT INTERACTIONS

In recent years, researchers and clinicians have expressed an increasing appreciation of the need to foster a positive emotional environment for parents and their infants in the NICU. This reflects the knowledge of what families need and their important role in promoting their infant's well-being. Interventions are being developed to assist families while in the NICU and during transition to home (Affleck, Tennen, Rowe, Roscher, & Walker, 1989; Norr, Nacion, & Abrahamson, 1989; Patteson & Barnard, 1990).

Some general guidelines for NICU health professionals working with parents to assist them in supportive parent-infant interactions include:

■ Teach parents to recognize infant states.
■ Encourage parents to interact with their infant in ways consistent with infant state and medical condition.
■ Help parents recognize signs of infant stimulus overload and when to stop providing any stimulation or interaction.
■ Provide guided instruction in interactions with infants.
■ Assist parents to understand the discrepancies between their infant's actual and expected behaviors.
■ Model and teach consoling and arousal techniques.
■ Identify infant feedback in parent-infant interactions.
■ Place parents in situations where they will experience positive or successful interactions with their infants.
■ Assist parents during interaction difficulties by pointing our infant state or positioning the infant for better interaction; modeling may by helpful.
■ Help parents to feel competent; recognize and praise appropriate and effective interventions.
■ Provide information on available support groups.
■ Keep parents informed about their infant's condition.

One intervention that NICU caregivers can use is to encourage parents to use formal and informal support systems. When support systems are minimal, staff can help parents to take advantage of available social services and parent support groups (Gottwald & Thurman, 1990). Some parents need to talk about their feeling with other parents of NICU infants.

Some NICUs assist family members who live long distances away with close living arrangements or living-in at hospital facilities. Often social services in intensive care nurseries help parents to locate resources such as babysitters to facilitate parent visitation.

NICU staff members can do many other things to assist parents to feel more confident with their infant. Listening may be the most helpful thing to do for parents of very ill infants. Providing parents with information about their infant's behaviors can help them respond appropriately. Parents need to know that although their baby may not be responding to them, they can sometimes help the baby by providing soothing stimulation such as talking softly or gently stroking, or simply letting the infant sleep. Staff can explain why infants should be protected from bright lights and noise. To guide parents in their individual approaches to their infant, staff can point out some of the baby's unique qualities. As the infant stabilizes, parents can be assisted to recognize their infant's individual behaviors and encouraged to become more actively involved in caregiving activities (Yoos, 1989).

Medical health providers in the neonatal intensive nursery must be sensitive to possible problems in the interaction process between parent and infant (Nici, 1989). While assessing the infant's cues for interaction readiness, NICU health professionals can assess parent behavior as well.

Effective interventions that facilitate early neonate supportive interactions must begin early in the neonatal intensive care nursery (VandenBerg, 1985). NICU caregivers, who are the infants' primary care providers during their hospital stay, can facilitate the development of positive parent-infant interactions in the following ways.

Encourage Parents

Staff can offer statements that help parents approach and interact with their infant. If the infant is too fragile for interactions staff can suggest that parents make a "visual visit" by just sitting by the bedside and looking at the baby. Statements such as "Look! She recognizes the sound of your voice!" or "He likes to look at your face" or "Now that you've tucked her in, she is sleeping quietly" acknowledge that parents are active agents for their infant. They encourage parents to interact with their infant.

Model Interventions

At times medical staff can model developmental interventions that promote parent-infant interactions. Modeling should be carried out in a way that does not undermine parent confidence. Shielding an infant's eyes from bright lights or positioning an infant with a pillow roll are techniques that help infants manage their environment. Demonstrate such techniques and point out the infant's responses to the intervention. Then assist the parent to try it. If the parent does try, provide positive feedback and encouragement. Take your time, use a step-by-step approach and be prepared to repeat what you do. Finally, do not forget that parents are probably watching everything you do. Consciously model good practice.

Reinforce Desired Behaviors

It is often unnecessary for professionals to teach parents how and when to interact with their infant. Too often opportunities are missed to give parents praise and credit for their appropriate interventions, caregiving, or interactions. Commenting on the effectiveness of the parents' actions on their infant's behaviors is powerful reinforcement for parents and probably just what they need to hear. Parents are learning that they are competent and important to their baby's well-being. For example, point out the baby's ability to calm down when swaddled by the parent.

Provide Information

Some parents will ask directly or indirectly for guidance. Instruction should be provided clearly and slowly to allow them to ask questions or practice. The message should be "Let's work together" rather than "I'm the expert." Look for opportunities to encourage or reinforce parents in the learning experience. Some NICUs provide written guidelines or illustrations for parents that provide instruction while minimizing the threatening aspects of instruction.

All of these methods assist parents to better understand their preterm infant and feel more comfortable in the unit setting. These are important components in promoting positive parent-preterm interactions.

Intervention support programs for parents have been found to help parents cope with the stressors associated with prematurity. One study reported that parents in the self-help intervention groups showed more involvement with their infants than did parents in control groups (Minde et al., 1980). Parents in the self-help groups also rated themselves as more confident in their parenting skills, and they continued to show more involvement with their infant 3 months after discharge.

A short-term, hospital-based teaching program for mothers of premature infants was implemented to study the program effects on subsequent mother-infant interventions (Harrison, Sherrod, Dunn, Olivet, & Jeong, 1991). Mothers of 32- to 36-week infants were randomly assigned to two experimental groups who received differential teaching instructions on infants' behavioral cues and a control group of mothers who received no teaching program. Mothers who participated in an instruction program that involved verbal instruction on the unique behavioral characteristics of their infants, observed an instructional videotape, and observed a behavioral assessment of their infant were significantly better able to assess their own infants' cues.

The experiences that parents have while in the NICU will influence the course of the their relationship with their infant. Providing an environment that both nurtures and encourages parent involvement with their infant is essential. Parents must feel welcomed and accepted by medical staff. They must have time to express their feelings and not be rushed to interact with their infant. NICU health professionals are in the unique position of providing support and reassurance to parents when they need it most.

■ SUMMARY

Parents of preterm infants may experience stress and anxiety as the result of their experience of having a premature infant. Not only is the premature birth traumatic, but the appearance and behavior of their preterm infant may cause mixed emotions. These feelings coupled with the infant's illness and the demands of the NICU environment may jeopardize early parent-preterm infant interactions.

Compared to healthy full-term infants, premature infants or very low birthweight newborns are less responsive and less capable of engaging in social interactions with their parents. The unavailability of the preterm infant as a social partner may alter the parent-infant partnership typical of full-term infants and their caregivers.

NICU health providers can structure interventions that support parents and infants and promote interactions appropriate to the infant's age, birthweight, and medical condition. Staff can provide information about the infant's behavior, reinforce appropriate interactions, and link parents to support networks.

■ REFERENCES

Affleck, G., Tennen, A., Rowe, J. Roscher, B., & Walker, L. (1989). Effects of formal support on mothers' adaptation to the hospital-to-home transition of high-risk infants: The benefits and costs of helping. *Child Development, 60*, 488–501.

Alfasi, G., Schwartz, F. A., Brake, S. C., Fifer, W. P., Fleischman, A. R., & Hofer, M. A. (1985). Mother-infant feeding interactions in preterm and full term infants. *Infant Behavior and Development, 8*, 167–80.

Als, H. (1979). Social interaction: Dynamic matrix for developing behavioral organization. *New Directions for Child Development, 4,* 21–39.

Bass, L. S. (1991). What do parents need when their infant is a patient in the NICU? *Neonatal Network, 10,* 25–33.

Brazelton, T. B. (1973). Neonatal Behavioral Assessment Scale. *Clinical Developmental Medicine,* No. 50.

Brooks-Gunn, J., Liaw, F. R., & Klebanov, P. K. (1992). Effects of early intervention on cognitive function of low birth weight preterm infants. *Journal of Pediatrics, 12,* 350–359.

Carey, W. B., & McDevitt, S. C. (1978). Revision of the Infant Temperament Questionnaire. *Pediatrics, 61,* 735–739.

Cohn, J. F., Matias, R., Tronick, E. Z., Lyons-Ruth, K., & Connell, D. (1986). Face-to-face interactions, spontaneous and structured, of mothers with depressive symptoms. In T. Field & E. Z. Tronick (Eds.), *Maternal depression and child development, New directions for child development* (pp. 31–46). San Francisco: Jossey-Bass.

Cohn, J. F., & Elmore, M. (1988). Effect of contingent changes in mothers' affective expression on the organization of behavior in 3 month old infants. *Infant Behavior and Development, 11,* 493–505.

Coll, C. T. G., & Meyer, E. C. (1993). The sociocultural context of infant development. In C. H. Zeanhah, Jr. (Ed.), *Handbook of infant mental health* (pp. 56–69). New York: Guilford.

Condon, W. S., & Sander, N. (1974). Neonate movement is synchronized with adult speech: Interactional participation and language acquisition. *Science, 183,* 99–101.

Craft, M. J., Wyatt, N., & Sandell, B. (1985). Behavior and feeding changes in siblings of hospitalized children. *Clinical Pediatrics, 24,* 374–378.

Crawford, J. W. (1982). Mother-infant interaction in premature and full-term infants. *Child Development, 53,* 957–962.

Crnic, K. A., Ragozin, A. S., Greenberg, M. T., Robinson, N. M., & Basham, R. B. (1983). Social interaction and developmental competence of preterm and full-term infants during the first year of life. *Child Development, 54,* 1199–1210.

Culp, R., Applebaum, M., Osofsky, J., & Levy, J. (1988). Adolescent and older mothers: Comparison between prenatal maternal variables and newborn interaction measures. *Infant Behavior and Development, 11,* 353–362.

DeCasper, A. J., & Fifer, W. P. (1980). Of human bonding: Newborns prefer their mother's voices. *Science, 208,* 1174–1176.

DiVitto, B., & Goldberg, S. (1979). The effects of newborn medical status on early parent-infant interaction. In T. M. Field (Ed.), *Infants born at risk: Behavior and development* (pp. 311–332). Jamaica, NY: SP Medical and Scientific Books.

Eckerman, C. O., & Oehler, J. M. (1992). Very low birthweight newborns and parents as early social partners. In S. L. Friedman & M. D. Sigman (Eds.), *The psychological development of low birthweight children: Annual advances in applied developmental psychology* (Vol. 6, pp. 91–123). Norwood, NJ: Ablex Publishing.

Eimas, P. D., Siqueland, E. R., Jusczyk, P., & Vigorito, J. (1971). Speech perception in infants. *Science, 171*, 303–306.

Emde, R. N., Gaensbauer, T. J., & Harmon, R. J. (1976). Emotional expression in infancy: A biological study. *Psychological Issues, 10*(1).

Epps, S. (1993). Labeling effects of infant health and parent demographics on nurses' ratings of preterm infant behavior. *Infant Mental Health Journal, 14*, 182–191.

Farnaroff, A. A., Kennell, J. H., & Klaus, M. H. (1972). Follow up of low birthweight infants: The predictive value of maternal visiting patterns. *Pediatrics, 49*, 287–290.

Field, T. (1977). Effects of early separation, interactive deficits and experimental manipulations on infant-mother face-to-face interactions. *Child Development, 48*, 763–771.

Field, T. (1982). Interaction coaching for high-risk infants and their parents. In H. A. Moss, K. Hess, & C. Swift (Eds.), *Early intervention programs for infants* (pp. 5–24). New York: Haworth Press.

Field, T. M. (1979). Interaction patterns of preterm and term infants. In T. M. Field, A. M. Sostek, S. Goldberg, & H. H. Shuman (Eds.), *Infants born at risk: Behavior and development* (pp. 333–361). New York: S. P. Medical & Scientific Books.

Fogel, A. (1991). *Infancy* (2nd ed.). St. Paul, MN: West Publishing.

Fogel, A., & Thelen, E. (1987). Development of early expressive and communicative action: Reinterpreting the evidence from a dynamic systems perspective. *Developmental Psychology, 23*, 747–761.

Freund, W. E. (1988). Prenatal attachment, the perinatal   continuum and the psychological side of neonatal intensive care. In P. Fedor-Freybergh & V. M. Vogel (Eds.), *Prenatal and perinatal psychology and medicine* (pp. 217–234). Park-Ridge, NJ: Parthenon.

Garcia-Coll, C. T., Emmons, L., Vohr, B. R., Ward, A. M., Brany, B. S., Shaul, P. W., Mayfield, S. R., & Oh, W. (1987). Behavioral responsiveness in preterm infants with intraventricular hemorrhage. *Pediatrics, 81*, 412–418.

Gennaro, S., Brooten, D., & Bakewell-Sacks, S. (1991). Post discharge services for low-birth-weight infants. *Journal of Obstetric, Gynecologic, and Neonatal Nursing, 20*, 29–36.

Goldberg, S. (1978). Prematurity: effects on parent-infant interactions. *Journal of Pediatric Psychology, 3*, 137–144.

Goldberg, S., & Divitto, B. A. (1983). *Born too soon.* San Francisco: W. H. Freeman.

Goldson, E. (1992). The neonatal intensive care unit: Premature infants and parents. *Infants and Young Children, 4*, 31–42.

Gottwald, S. R., & Thurman, S. K. (1990). Parent-infant interaction in neonatal intensive care units: Implications for research and service delivery. *Infants and Young Children, 2*, 1–9.

Griffin, T. (1990). Nurse barriers to parenting in the special care nursery. *Journal of Perinatal Nursing, 4*, 56–67.

Gustafson, G. E., & Harris, K. L. (1990). Women's responses to young infants' cries. *Developmental Psychology, 26*, 144–152.

Harrison, L., Sherrod, R. A., Dunn, L., Olivet, L., & Jeong, J. (1991). Effects of hospital-based instruction on interactions between parents and preterm infants. *Neonatal Network, 9,* 27–33.

Hayes, M. J., & Ensher, G. L. (1994). Intervening in intensive care nurseries. In G. L. Ensher & D. A. Clark (Eds.), *Newborns at risk* (pp. 227–248). Gaithersburg, MD: Aspen.

Jarvis, P. A., Myers, B. J., & Creasey, G. L. (1989). The effects of infants' illness on mothers' interactions with prematures at 4 and 8 months. *Infant Behavior and Development, 12,* 25–35.

Klaus, M. H., & Robertson, M. O. (1982). *Birth, interaction and attachment.* Skillman, NJ: John & Johnson.

Lawhon, G. (1986). Management of stress in premature infants. In D. J. Angelini, C. M. Whelan-Knapp, & M. Gibes (Eds.), *Perinatal/neonatal nursing: A clinical handbook* (pp. 319–328). Boston: Blackwell Scientific Publications.

Lee, S. K., Penner, P. L., & Cox, M. (1991). Impact of very low birthweight infants on the family and its relationship to parental attitudes. *Pediatrics, 88,* 105–109.

Lester, B. M., Emory, E. K., Hoffman, S. L., & Eitzman, D. V. (1976). A multivariant study of the effects of high-risk factors on performance on the Brazelton Neonatal Assessment Scales. *Child Development, 47,* 515–517.

Lester, B. M., Hoffan, J., & Brazelton, T. B. (1985). The rhythm structure of mother interaction in term and preterm infants. *Child Development, 56,* 15–27.

Levy-Shiff, R., Hoffman, M. A., Mogilner, S., Levinger, S., & Mogilner, M. B. (1990). Fathers' hospital visits to their preterm infants as a predictor of father-infant relationship and infant development. *Pediatrics, 86,* 289–293.

Levy-Shiff, R., Sharir, H., & Mogilner, M. B. (1989). Mother-and father-preterm infant relationship in the hospital preterm nursery. *Child Development, 60,* 93–102.

Lewis, M., Bendersky, M., Koons, A., Hegyi, T., Hiatt, M., Ostfield, B., & Rosenfield, D. (1991). Visitation to a neonatal intensive care unit. *Pediatrics, 88,* 795–800.

Macey, T. J., Harmon, R. J., & Easterbrooks, M. A. (1987). Impact of premature birth of the infant in the family. *Journal of Consulting and Clinical Psychology, 55,* 846–852.

Macfarlane, A. (1975). Olfaction in the development of social preferences in the human neonate. In CIBA Foundation Symposium (Ed.), *Parent-infant interaction* (pp. 103–117). New York: Elsevier.

Marton, P., Minde, K., & Perrotta, M. (1981). The role of father for the infant at risk. *American Journal of Orthopsychiatry, 51,* 672–679.

Maurer, D. C., & Maurer, C. (1988). *The world of the newborn.* New York: Basic Books.

McCluskey-Fawcett, K., O'Brien, M., Robinson, P., & Asay, J. H. (1992). Early transition for the parents of premature infants: Implications for interventions. *Infant Mental Health Journal, 13,* 147–156.

McGehee, L. J., & Eckerman, C. O. (1983). The preterm infant as a social partner: Responsive but unreadable. *Infant Behavior and Development, 6,* 461–470.

McHaffie, H. E. (1992). Social support in the neonatal intensive care unit. *Journal of Advanced Nursing, 17*, 279–287.

Meltzoff, A., & Moore, W. K. (1977). Imitation of facial and manual gestures by human neonates. *Science, 198*, 75–78.

Meltzoff, A., & Moore, W. K. (1989). Imitation in newborn infants: Exploring the range of gestures imitated and the underlying mechanisms. *Developmental Psychology, 25*, 954–962.

Miller, M. D., & Ottinger, D. R. (1986). Influence of labeling on ratings of infant behavior. A prematurity prejudice. *Journal of Pediatric Psychology, 11*, 561–572.

Minde, K. (1992). The social and emotional development of low-birthweight infants and their families up to age 4. In S. L. Friedman & M. D. Sigman (Eds.), *The psychological development of low birthweight children: Annual advances in developmental psychology* (Vol. 1, pp. 157–185). Norwood, NJ: Ablex Publishing.

Minde, K. (1993). Prematurity and serious medical illness in infancy: Implications for development and intervention. In C. H. Zeanah, Jr. (Ed.), *Handbook of infant mental health* (pp. 87–105). New York: Guilford.

Minde, K., Perrotta, M., & Marton, P. (1985). Maternal caretaking and play with full term and premature infants. *Journal of Child Psychology and Psychiatry, 26*, 231–244.

Minde, K., Shosenberg, N., Marton, P., Thompson, J., Ripley, J., & Burns, S. (1980). Self-help groups in a premature nursery—A controlled evaluation. *Journal of Pediatrics, 96*, 933–940.

Minde, K. K., Trehub, S., Corte, C., Boukydis, C., Celhoffer, L., & Marton, P. (1978). Mother-child relationships in the premature nursery. *Pediatrics, 61*, 373–389.

Minde, K., Whitelaw, A., Brown, J., & Fitzhardinge, P. (1983). Effect of neonatal complications in premature infants on early parent-infant interaction. *Developmental Medicine and Child Neurology, 25*, 763—75.

Nici, J. (1989). Parent-infant interaction. In C. J. Semmler (Ed.), *A guide to care and management of very low birthweight infants: A team approach* (pp. 32–50). Tucson, AZ: Therapy Skill Builders.

Norr, K. F., Nacion, K. W., & Abrahamson, R. (1989). Early discharge with home follow-up: Impacts on low-income mothers and infants. *Journal of Obstetric, Gynecologic, and Neonatal Nursing, 18*, 138–141.

Paludetto, R., Dell'Antonio, A. M., DeCurtis, M., DeVito, P., & Devito, G. (1984). Madre-neonato: Evoluzione del rapporto in un reparto di patologia neonatale aperto ai genitori. Confronto con un reparto tradizionale. *Eta Evolutiva, 19*, 35–40.

Parker, S. J., Zahn, L. K., Cole, J. G., & Brecht, M. (1992). Outcome after developmental intervention in the neonatal intensive care unit for mothers of preterm infant with low socioeconomic status. *Journal of Pediatrics, 120*, 780–785.

Patteson, D. M., & Barnard, K. E. (1990). Parenting of low birth weight infants: A review of issues and interventions. *Infant Mental Health, 11*, 37–56.

Perlman, N. B., Freedman, J. L. Abramovitch, R., Whyte, H., Kirpalam, H., & Perlman, M. (1991). Information needs of parents of sick neonates. *Pediatrics, 88*, 512–518.

Plaas, K. M. (1994). The evolution of parental roles in the NICU. *Neonatal Network, 13*, 31–33.

Prechtl, H. F. R., Fargel, J. W., Weinmann, H. M., & Bakker, H. T. (1979). Postures, motility and respiration of low-risk preterm infants. *Developmental Medicine and Child Neurology, 21*, 3–27.

Rose, S. A. (1983). Behavioral and psychophysiological sequelae of preterm birth: The neonatal period. In T. Field & A. Sostek (Eds.), *Infants born at risk: Physiological, perceptual and cognitive processes* (pp. 45–67). New York: Grune & Stratton.

Rosenfield, A. G. (1980). Visiting the intensive care nursery. *Child Development, 51*, 939–941.

Rushton, C. H. (1990). Strategies for family-centered care in the critical care setting. *Pediatric Nursing, 16*, 195–199.

Schwab, F., Tolbert, B., Bagnuto, S., & Meisels, M. J. (1983). Sibling visits in a neonatal intensive care unit. *Pediatrics, 7*, 835–838.

Spungen, L. B., & Farran, A. C. (1986). Effect of intensive care unit exposure on temperament in low birth weight preterm infants. *Journal of Developmental and Behavioral Pediatrics, 7*, 288–292.

Stern, D. (1982). Mother and infants: The early transmission of affect. In M. H. Klaus & M. O. Robertson (Eds.), *Birth, interaction and attachment* (pp. 43–50). Skillman, NJ: Johnson & Johnson.

Stern, M., & Hildebrandt, K. A. (1984). Prematurity stereotype: Effects of labeling on adults' perception of infants. *Developmental Psychology, 20*, 360–362.

Stern, M., & Hildebrant, K. A. (1986). Prematurity stereotyping: Effects on mother-infant interaction. *Child Development, 57*, 308–315.

Stern, M., & Karraker, K. H. (1988). Prematurity stereotyping by mothers of premature infants. *Journal of Pediatric Psychology, 13*, 255–263.

Stern, M., & Karraker, K. H. (1990). The prematurity stereotype: Empirical evidence and implications for practice. *Infant Mental Health Journal, 11*, 3–11.

Thoman, E. B., & Browder, S. (1987). *Born dancing.* New York: Harper & Row.

Thomas, A., & Chess, S. (1977). *Temperament and development.* New York: Brunner-Mazel.

Thurman, S. K., & Korteland, C. (1987). The behavior of mothers and fathers toward their infants during neonatal intensive care visits. *Children's Health Care, 18*, 247–251.

Tinsley, B., & Parke, R. (1983). The person-environment relationship: Lessons from families with preterm infants. In D. Magnusson & V. Allen (Eds.), *Human Development: An interactional perspective* (pp. 93–110). New York: Academic Press.

VandenBerg, K. (1985). Revising the traditional model: An individualized approach to developmental interventions in the intensive care nursery. *Neonatal Network, 3*(5), 32–38.

Washington, J., Minde, K., & Goldberg, S. (1986). Temperament in preterm infants: Style and stability. *Journal of the American Academy of Child Psychiatry, 25,* 493–502.

Wilfong, E. W., Saylor, C., & Elksnin, N. (1991). Influence on responsiveness: Interaction between mothers and their premature infants. *Infant Mental Health Journal, 12,* 31–40.

Yoos, L. (1989). Applying research in practice: Parenting the premature infant. *Applied Nursing Research, 2,* 30–34.

Zeskind, P. S., & Lester, B. M. (1978). Acoustic features of auditory perceptions of the cries of newborns with prenatal complications. *Child Development, 49,* 580–589.

Zeskind, P. S., & Lester, B. M. (1981). Analysis of cry features in newborns with differential fetal growth. *Child Development, 52,* 207–212.

Zeskind, P. S., & Iacino, R. (1984). Effects of maternal visitation to preterm infants in the neonatal intensive care unit. *Child Development, 55,* 1887–1893.

■ CHAPTER 8

Family Reactions to Premature Birth

"Fasten your seat belts, we are in
for a bumpy ride."
Bette Davis in All About Eve

■ INTRODUCTION

The birth of a premature infant is a traumatic event, a bumpy ride, in any family's life. The ideal pregnancy is conceived out of dreams and is filled with hope, but an infant who is born "too soon" may threaten a family's dream and frustrate the realization of a family's hopes. For most parents a premature birth is not the way a pregnancy is supposed to turn out. It is important that we understand the family's loss and the potential crisis a high risk birth creates. Parents, whoever they may be, find that they are out of their league and swimming in very deep water. This chapter will focus on the family experience, identify psychological and social needs of these families, and examine the variety of families in the premature nursery. In the following chapter we will focus attention on appropriate family interventions and ways to make NICUs more family-centered.

Babies who come into the world too soon inevitably find their way to a Neonatal Intensive Care Unit (NICU), whose acronym is sometimes pronounced as NICKYOU (Mehren, 1991). NICUs have been likened to a landed spacecraft, a MASH Unit for infants, and a shrine to high technology. The high-technology hospital nursery is a bright, noisy, sometimes cluttered, action packed, trauma center where high-risk infants are saved by professionals who use the latest advances of science and medicine. It is a place where miracles happen that only a decade ago were beyond our imagination. The medical advances and the rate of change has been phenomenal.

A NICU serving 50 babies can have up to 150 employees staffing that unit 24 hours a day, 7 days a week, every week. Among the people who staff these units are neonatologists, attendings, surgeons, residents, RNs, LPNs, occupational therapists, respiratory therapists, physical therapists, nurses, parent educators, social workers, psychologists, and entry and discharge personnel.

Parents and families enter this remarkable environment because it is where their premature infants are being treated. This might be for a few days. It could be for several months, and for some, it could be years. These parents arrive in the NICU like foreigners in a strange land. Everything seems out of proportion. The activities and the language are unfamiliar. The atmosphere sends the message that only highly skilled people enter here. A metaphor employed by some families is that they had airline tickets to lovely Seattle, Washington, but their plane landed in Bosnia during the civil war. Dedicated staff, who have adjusted and adapted to this unique environment, sometimes forget just how difficult a NICU can be for families.

The trauma of a premature birth and the hospitalization of premature infants is highly stressful for families in part because patterns of normal parenting and parent-infant interactions are disrupted (Goldberger, 1987). Families feel helpless and experience a loss of control (Affleck, Tennen, Allen, & Rowe, 1986). Learning to cope with the many stressors associated with caring for a preterm baby is added to whatever burdens and stressors may already exist in the lives of these families. The critical challenge this presents to even the most intact family is readily apparent. What happens to an already dysfunctional family is difficult to understand.

■ FAMILY DIFFERENCES

Families whose infants are placed in a NICU come from a wide variety of backgrounds and experiences. Although the young and the poor are disproportionately represented in the population, virtually all classes and ethnic groups, married and unmarried, are involved (Johnson, 1983). Some of the mothers have had no prenatal care. Others have been seeing physicians regularly because their pregnancy was known to have difficulties or potential problems. Still others have had no warning that there might be anything at all unusual in the birth.

Parent types vary, and there is an even wider range of responses to this critical event in a family's life. Some parents know a great deal about the medical facts surrounding the anticipated birth, while others cannot explain the biological facts of pregnancy. There are mothers who feel alone and isolated and mothers who have extended families and large support groups. Some parents have other children at home or this may be their first born. They may seek information and assistance on their own or they might rely totally on the NICU staff for guidance. This pregnancy might be the fulfillment of a couple's dream or it might be a nightmare. A woman might have a husband, several boyfriends, or no one at all. There are parents ready to be totally involved in the care and monitoring of their child (see Figure 8–1) and others who must be brought into caregiving activities gradually. Numerous factors interact in this critical experience. How well a family does involves several important factors: its ability to adapt to the unusual and challenging intensive care environment (Briggs, 1985; Johnson, 1983), the medical condition of the infant (Littman, 1979), the families' coping skills under stress (Affleck, Tennen, McGrade, & Katzan, 1985), and the level of difficulty in obtaining support from significant others and medical staff (Crnic, Greenberg, & Slough, 1986).

Because of the wide range of families and parents, it is not accurate or useful to generalize about them. It is a mistake and a disservice to approach families as if "one size fits all." To be most helpful to parents, time must be spent finding out about some of the details of their world, and an assessment should be made of each family's needs

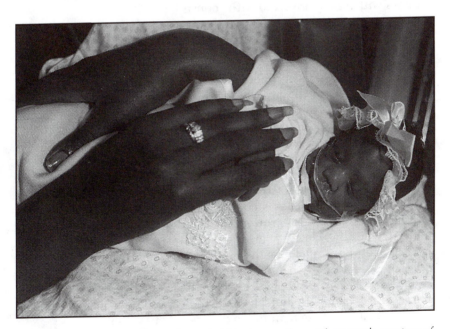

FIGURE 8–1. A preterm infant being held by her mother.. (Photograph courtesy of Children's Hospital of Buffalo Department of Medical Photography.)

(Bailey & Simeonsson, 1988). Although this is sometimes difficult to achieve, it is important for NICU staff to see each family as distinct in order not to prejudge and categorize people unfairly (Hughes, McCollum, Sheftel, & Sanchez, 1994). It is as important for staff to assess parent psychosocial needs as it is for staff to assess infant cues, attentional states, and needs (Johnson, 1979).

Staff need to remain sensitive to how difficult the NICU environment is to the family. The NICU staff must interpret the infant's medical condition and the parameters for parent intervention, assess the coping skills of the parent and the limits they might have for involvement with their infant, and determine the level of support the parent(s) presently has and the amount of support the parent(s) might need from the staff and others.

Each parent brings a different set of experiences and expectations to the NICU. Sometimes the staff is tempted to give most of their time to the most capable and temperamentally easy parents. As a result, the parents who need the most assistance may receive very little. If parents are stereotyped and judged before attempts are made to involve them with their infant, the result may be little parental involvement. Helping create the right match between parents and their infants increases the likelihood that eventually the parents will become involved with their infant.

■ CATEGORIZING FAMILIES

Like most of us, health professionals often relate better with people they think are like themselves. Middle-class NICU staff are more likely to feel comfortable with middle-class, intact families. It is not uncommon to see two or three nurses interacting with an intact family while a young, minority, single mother is left alone with her infant.

NICU staff members appear to have developed a system of categorizing the NICU infant population. For example, at first an infant might be called a baby, a fetus, or a nonviable. Later it might be called a good baby or a sick baby; and still later it might be referred to as a "chronic," a "feeder," a "grower," or a "graduate." Whatever term is used, it typically relates to a set of expectations and predictions that medical staff have made for the baby. To a certain extent, these labels set the stage for how the staff members expect to relate to the infant (Epps, 1993). They also help determine the extent of attachment to the infant. For example, if nurses think that an infant will not make it, they are more likely to maintain a distance (Lopez, 1983).

A similar process occurs with families. Staff members may judge parents to be viable or nonviable, valued or devalued, good, not so good, or bad. Some parents are thought to have potential and to be cooperative, while others are viewed as difficult or problematic. In certain nurseries, families are viewed as visitors, workers, or patients. Staff members prefer that families assume a visitor's role because visitors observe proper limits. Especially good visitors may graduate to a worker role if the nurse deems it appropriate. But if a family crosses limits set by staff, they may be assigned a patient role, that is, they are perceived as problems (Griffin, 1990). These examples are not hard-and-fast categories. Sometimes even good parents become a problem, for instance when they think nurses are not doing enough for their infant. And a "bad" parent who, for example, comes through for the baby after some difficult periods of grieving may be elevated to a more positive role. Health professionals need to remain nonjudgemental and assist in positive parental involvement.

Although there are differences across the country and from nursery to nursery, NICU medical staff often use some of the following characteristics to categorize parents:

Valued Parents	**Devalued Parents**
Reasonable income	Limited finances
Intelligent	Uneducated or too smart
Visits often	Visits too little or too much
Couples	Single or with several men
Over 21	Too young or too old
Has support people	Has few social supports
Shows understanding	Unresponsive or unrealistic
Assertive	Passive or aggressive
Interacts with infant	Withdrawn from infant
Learns skills	Does not manage new skills
Background similar to staff	Different background and
Easy to communicate with	culture
Gives and receives praise	Difficult to talk with
	Has difficulty giving and
	receiving praise

Bogden, Brown, and Foster (1982) identified some of the ways a nursing staff forms judgments about parents. When asked to define a well-adjusted or a poorly adjusted parent, they followed a pattern similar to the one outlined above.

The "good" parents ask good questions, understand the seriousness of the situation, and tolerate ambiguity in diagnosis and prognosis. They appreciate staff and conform to unit rules and schedules. They visit regularly, show interest, telephone regularly, and react appropriately to reports on their infant's condition. They attach themselves to their infant and show potential as care providers.

"Poor" parents, however, do few or none of the above. If they visit at all, it is brief, and they keep a distance from staff and child. They do not appear to cope well and show little potential to become adequate caregivers (Bogden et al., 1982).

Although practices such as these are common, Bogden et al. (1982) warn us that such judgments tend to be made too quickly and are based on limited information, "short observations," "limited or no conversation," and "second-hand reporting." Because judgments negatively impact on their work with families, NICU health professionals need to take more time and care in labeling or attempt to not label at all.

■ YOU DON'T UNDERSTAND

Families in a NICU commonly feel that other people do not understand their plight. The birth of a premature infant is so different from normal expectations that it throws many parents into a tailspin. Some describe it as a dizzying experience. Many feel like victims in an event that is happening to them rather than with them. Most parents of medically fragile newborns describe the experience as emotionally wrenching.

Parents often describe their underlying emotional experience as being out of control (Affleck, Tennen, Rowe, & Higgins, 1990). They say that the experience is so disorienting that it causes them to feel that others cannot possibly understand. Their taken-for-granted view of an orderly world is shaken; assumptions about the way life is supposed to be are thrown into question; the idea of being able to make orderly plans, predict events within reason, and set meaningful goals is challenged. Many parents feel alone in this experience.

Most families of premature infants experience both a primary loss and a range of emotions referred to as grief (Gardner & Merenstein, 1986). Primary loss results from the parents' feeling that they have lost the normal infant they were supposed to have (Sammons & Lewis, 1985). The baby of the parents' dreams is gone; their infant was born too soon, is fragile, too small, underdeveloped, and may not live. If the baby does live, what kind of problems will the child and the family face?

Families of preterm infants face enormous readjustments in their thinking, feelings, and actions (Taylor & Hall, 1979). The experience can raise questions about one's values and beliefs, weaken self-esteem, and challenge the understanding of purpose in life. Relationships, marriages, and families tend to suffer great disequilibrium during this time. Losses are often difficult to talk about because they are losses connected to expectations of a full-term delivery. What can we say about a lost dream? Our understanding of this question may help us get closer to the parent experience. A story may help us understand what certain parents are experiencing in this situation.

A geni escaped from her bottle because a more powerful geni wanted to hurt her. She escaped into the laboratory of a great scientist whom she begged to protect her. They were discussing strategy when the powerful geni appeared and began to punish, beat, and seriously threaten the escaped geni. In desperation the scientist used a magic formula that made the enemy disappear.

In absolute gratitude the now safe geni said to the scientist, "You have saved my life. Name three wishes and I will grant them to you." The scientist requested that the laboratory be expanded with needed equipment for greater work. "Of course, your wish is granted, but your request is so small."

For the second wish the scientist asked for able assistants to help with the work. "Of course I will grant you however many assistants you want, but you ask for so little. You are frustrating me with your requests. Take care that you make good use of your last request."

Unable to contain his curiosity any longer, the scientist asked, "I would like to know how you felt when the other geni was threatening your life?" The geni became offended, saying, "How dare you ask about a geni's feelings? The punishment for this insult shall be death."

The geni had the scientist arrested and sentenced to die in the morning by hanging. During the night, the scientist wept for the mistake and feared for the morning. The terror increased as they came to the place of execution to face the hangman. The rope was tightened around the scientist's neck before the walk down the ten foot plank was begun.

The scientist walked step by terrified step toward the end of the plank when the hangman shouted, "Stop!" They loosened and removed the rope and placed a note in the scientist's hand. Gradually his eyes opened and his body relaxed enough to read the note. It said, "You wanted to know how I felt when I was threatened by the other geni. Now you know."

The geni knew that some things in life are beyond words. There are life events that need to be experienced before they can be fully understood. Only by placing the scientist's life in a similar life-threatening situation would the scientist be able to "know" and feel the geni's terror.

Many grieving parents feel like the geni in the story. They feel that their isolation, terror, fear, and the threat they experience can only be understood by someone in a similar circumstance. It is quite common for parents to feel that others cannot possibly know what it feels like to experience this loss (Mehren, 1991).

Such feelings may result in parents distancing themselves from the people about them. It can occur between parents and their friends, neighbors, and other members of their families. Parents may even distance themselves from the most caring and understanding professional. It can happen even if all the right things are being done for the infant and parents. It happens because these parents have intense and powerful experiences with loss. Fortunately, such distancing does not occur with all parents and most find ways to overcome potential barriers in their relationship with health professionals (Affleck, Tennen, & Rowe, 1991; Griffin, 1990).

Because of the strong possibility of negative consequences, it is important to identify common emotional responses to a primary loss in a person's life. All losses are not equal and no two persons will respond exactly alike; however, there are common threads in the human experience. Recognizing and understanding normal reactions to loss are key to understanding the family experience in the NICU. Parents have lost their anticipated normal full-term baby. Now they have a fragile baby who is not with them but is being cared for by the NICU staff. Their anticipated roles as new parents also are lost. Mothers are asked to assume a new, strange, sometimes alien form of motherhood, and fathers are expected to undertake a difficult and challenging form of parenting (Goldberg & Divito, 1983).

In retrospective studies several themes tend to occur for a majority of families. Painful memories live at the surface and are easily recalled. Some of the memories relate to the place. "I remember the fear and terror in the pit of my stomach and the sights and sounds of that place." Some relate to the infant. "Will my baby live or die? Which is better?" Parents also ask: "Whose baby is it? My baby is not with me. The NICU has our baby." Loss of control is very common. "I have memories of feeling that everything is out of my hands. That nothing I do will make any difference. I am powerless in this circumstance." There is also the inevitable comparison with staff. "The NICU professionals are more competent than we mere parents. It is easier to leave our baby in the hands of the staff" (McCauley & McCauley, 1987).

Such reports are among the most commonly mentioned difficulties that parents connect with their NICU experience. Although such experiences are probably inevitable, health professionals need to remember that it is possible to ease such difficulties. Efforts to help families make adjustments to this difficult situation pay dividends for the family, for the baby, and for health professionals.

■ THE ROLLER COASTER

A child is conceived. As the child grows in the womb, a new phase of a life begins and gradually changes the mother and father to be. Will it be a boy or girl? Will the baby be a daughter, a new woman in the family carrying hopes and dreams? or a son, a new man in the family bearing fulfillment and promise? Changes are anticipated; joys and frustrations are shared, and the future already takes shape. But when the birthday comes it is not with joy but with fear. Instead of fanfare and celebration, there is bewilderment and frustration. The baby was born 10 weeks too early. This mother and father have begun a new journey.

NICU parent graduates have a common bond. They call it the roller coaster experience. Regardless of their place and position in life, whoever they may be, whatever their social mobility, parents whose infants require intensive care experience an emotional roller coaster ride. The length and severity of the ride depends upon the infant's medical condition, the length of stay in intensive care, the support that parents receive from others, and the coping skills of the parents.

In a sense the NICU is an equal opportunity facility. Parents are leveled in this place of machines where every conversation is public, emotions are difficult to express or hide, and one's infant is exposed to scrutiny and comparison. The college graduate and the school dropout, the suburban housewife and the single-parent inner-city adolescent, and the businessman and the adolescent father are equally humbled in this shrine to the best that medicine and science can create.

NICU parents often have a difficult time with people outside the hospital; included are family, friends, and colleagues. The parents' ups and downs, their optimism and despair, the rapid shifting through the range of emotions, and the intensity of the experience are all involved. They know they are having difficulty sorting it all out and cannot hope to have outsiders understand. It may be one of the reasons why it sometimes takes time for parents to open up to hospital staff and why some parents first look to other parents in the same situation. (Mehren, 1991).

Every parent who has been in a NICU understands the emotional roller coaster. It comes with conflicting interpretations of their baby's condition; it happens each time the infant's medical condition changes, up or down, and it comes with shift changes and nurse changes. Some parents will be in denial and cling to hope against a poor prognosis; others will want to give up despite the progress and gains of their infant. One day they feel this could not be happening to them; the next day they know the challenge is theirs. Parents and staff need to know that such emotional swings are normal and to be expected in this crisis situation (Wyly & Allen, 1990).

In the following chapter we will discuss interventions that assist parents to cope with this emotional crisis.

■ THE GRIEVING PROCESS

Grieving is a process of coming to terms with loss. Parents who have not anticipated an early birth have considerable adjusting to do. Grief is a response to loss, no matter how insignificant or intense. For many parents grief is a response to the stress of the unexpected early birth of their child (Hummel & Eastman, 1991).

Parents who have everything planned down to the day they would bring their perfect baby home may need considerable time and support to adapt to a prematurely born infant. Parents who do not have high expectations for their own lives, as well as parents who do have great expectations, are likely to feel incompetent and experience low self-esteem and failure when their infant is born prematurely. New parents who feel deprived of their traditional roles as parents are likely to feel empty. The infant's medical setbacks can cause anxiety for parents. In each instance, parents grieve.

People grieve the loss of their dreams. What dreams are being broken for the couple who had everything just right, and then . . .; for the couple who were just getting it together, and then . . .; for the adolescent who did not want to be pregnant, and then . . .? Because so much is happening in the NICU, the staff may overlook parents and their loss. Professionals may think the baby is not that sick or only mildly disabled, while parents are devastated because this has happened to their child. What happens is that professionals and parents look at the experience from different perspectives (Rosenthal, Marscall, MacPherson, & French, 1980).

Grieving begins with the loss of a dream. Human beings are directed in large part by dreams and expectations. Parents of premature infants have lost the dream of a normal healthy infant. What was that dream? In what way has reality shattered the dream? Who was the child supposed to be before its premature birth? Learning what parents' dreams were will help NICU health professionals to anticipate parents' reaction to loss.

Although descriptions of grief reactions are common in literature, drama, and theater, clinical studies of the grief process have a fairly short history. One of the first systematic studies was done by Lindemann, who studied survivors of World War II and the Coconut Grove fire in Boston (Lindemann 1944). He concluded that the survivors experienced feelings and reactions similar to those following the loss of a loved one. Survivors initially felt shock, numbness, disbelief. Later they felt guilty and depressed. Some experienced chronic sadness. Parents and family members report similar reactions to a miscarriage, newborn's death, premature birth, infant with disabilities, and infant born at risk (Hynan, 1986).

Kubler-Ross (1969), building on the work of Lindemann, familiarized people with the grieving process. The contribution of her work is enormous. Kubler-Ross identified five stages of grief: denial, anger, bargaining, depression, and acceptance. According to Kubler-Ross, these grief stages relate both to the dying person and to those anticipating the person's death, and they may or may not occur in an orderly, linear sequence. Working through grief refers to the survivor coming to terms with the stages of grief.

However, we need to be careful because erroneous assumptions and oversimplifications have accompanied Kubler-Ross's model. For example, some concluded that a grieving person moves from one stage to another, from denial through acceptance, until the grief process is complete. In fact, not everyone experiences any or all of the grief stages. Some do not recover from grief for years or may never complete the grieving process. This often is the case for parents who experience difficulties with the birth of their child (Cole, 1987). Some parents never accept their loss. Others report thinking they have reached acceptance only to return to a stage they think they have left. This often occurs when infants are unable to reach an appropriate milestone in their development. There are parents who are characterized as in chronic sorrow over the personal loss they have not been able to accept or resolve (Hummel & Eastman, 1991).

At the birth of a premature or high-risk infant, some parents feel a primary loss that results in disorientation and tremendous sadness (Schiff, 1977). It is one of the most serious stressors a person can experience. How an individual deals with this crisis is called grief work or process. NICU parents do not experience an orderly progressive sequence of grief steps, instead they experience what is referred to as emotional states (Wyly & Allen, 1990). This is a dynamic, often rapidly changing process from one state to another.

"Parent states" refers to a set of emotional reactions that occur when parents experience personal loss. Parents report that they feel shock and sheer terror during the early stages of a premature birth. Later they tend to experience a range of emotions including guilt, anger, and jealousy. A common emotional state is guilt and self-blaming: "I caused my child's problems. I know how I did it." Sometimes it may be, "It's all your fault." Anger and guilt about the premature birth may come and go for many years. It is not unusual for depression and low self-esteem to recur over time (Benfield, Leib, & Reuter, 1976).

Individuals cope with their grief in individual ways, influenced by background, education, culture, religion, family, and friends. Reactions to grief vary greatly. Husbands and wives are not likely to cope with having an infant in the NICU in the same way. A mature middle-class family's coping will likely differ from the coping of an inner-city adolescent. NICU staff must look for differences and learn to assess the different coping styles that parents will use.

■ PARENT STATES

We prefer the use of emotional states rather than stages because it more accurately describes the dynamic process most parents experience (Wyly & Allen, 1990). Like their premature infants who often transition quickly from one behavioral state to another, parents can move rapidly in and out of emotional states. Although considerable movement across emotions occurs for many parents, many parents stay in shock or depression for long periods of time.

A dynamic, ever-changing process is much more helpful to understanding parents than the assumption that parents will go through a particular fixed set of stages. We find that health professionals have an intuitive understanding of the grieving process and are very receptive to approaching emotional states as a dynamic, ever-changing process.

The grief work parents must do involves a process of encountering and working through intense emotional states. In the fishbowl-like environment of the NICU this is difficult to do, but, remarkably, it happens every day. It is a natural, normal process assisted by allowing grieving persons to experience and talk about their feelings related to their loss.

When this occurs in a caring context it is a powerful and memorable event. Parents have vivid memories of the first person they feel really understood what they were experiencing. "I remember the nurse who told me how tough this was going to be." "I remember the parent who came up and touched and comforted me with her few words." "I recall the nurse who said, 'You are having a hard time today,' and then let me talk."

The following are brief descriptions of the parent states likely to be seen in the NICU (Benfield et al., 1976). We have identified the emotional state, the nonverbal cues you might see and the feelings. Included also are interventions designed to help staff communicate with families. A wide range of interventions and techniques to support families will be discussed in Chapter 9.

The Parent States

Shock or Terror

The initial impact of the unexpected early arrival of their premature infant places many parents in a state of shock or terror. The infant is often moved to another part of the hospital or to a larger regional hospital better equipped to serve the needs of the neonate. Parents report feeling overwhelmed, distraught and disorganized (Benfield et al., 1976; Briggs, 1985; Hummel & Eastman, 1991). They are unable to focus, concentrate, or process much information, and sometimes they make rash decisions due to this emotional state. Often they sign papers or engage in conversations they cannot remember later.

Signs and cues: Glazed look, overwhelmed and dazed, distraught and disorganized, lacking focus or concentration, unable to process information, blank expression, poor eye contact, loss of routines, unkempt appearance, forgetfulness, absentmindedness

Feelings: Empty, out of control, futility, overwhelmed, incompetent

Underlying statements: "This is all too much for me." "This is the straw that broke my back."

Interventions: Greet parents when they first enter the nursery, and try to make them comfortable. Use a quiet, soft voice and silence. Do not overwhelm them with information, but use positive words about the infant. Provide simple guidance and suggestions: "You can watch or help if you like"; or "Take a break for a while." Engage in small talk only if the parents seem willing. Explain clearly what you need to do with the infant. Involve support people whenever possible. Keep serious questions at a minimum.

Fear

Parents can be so blinded by fear that they are unable to make any attachment to their infant. They feel too vulnerable. Often they show symptoms of fear until they are certain that their infant is getting better. Unlike anxiety, which is about our total life, fear has an object and can change when the object of fear is removed or changed.

Signs and cues: Detachment, distancing, frozen robot-like motions, tense facial expression, darting eyes, avoidance, rapid speech, topic changing, avoiding the infant, leaving early, failure to visit

Feelings: Vulnerable, fragile, weak, incompetent, not wanting to get attached

Underlying statements: "My baby will suffer and maybe die." "I can't do this." "It is going to hurt too much." "I don't have what it takes."

Interventions: Acknowledge that we are all vulnerable. Pain, fear, and hurt are part of our fragile lives. Let parents know that you are trying to understand their fear. Do not pressure them. Talk gently; if you and they feel comfortable, touch them gently. Position yourself close to them if possible. Talk positively about the infant, but be realistic about the fears. Stop talking if parents appear to be overwhelmed; you can be silent for a while and still show that you are supportive. Allow parents to cry. If you leave them, let them know when you are coming back. Talk plainly and simply about the things you are doing with the infant.

Guilt

Guilt is nearly inevitable among parents whose infants are in an intensive care nursery. Whether or not a basis for guilt can be identified, many parents feel responsible for their infant's condition. It is common for a parent to think if only they had done something differently, this would not have happened. The following are some of the different ways parents might express their guilt.

1. It is all my fault. I caused my child's problem, and I know how I did it. (I used drugs; I abused myself; we went to the wrong physician...).
2. This is punishment for something that I thought, felt, said, or did. Many times I thought, "I wish I were not having this child."
3. Good things happen to good people, bad things happen to bad people. Therefore, I must be bad.
4. "What should we have done differently?" "Why have we been singled out?" These thoughts inevitably reflect feelings of guilt.

Guilt accompanies any major life loss. Guilt is present whether or not a person is responsible for a problem. Parents in the NICU often feel guilty over their inability to care for their vulnerable infants (Whetsell & Larrabee, 1988).

Signs and cues: Dejection, blaming self, little eye contact, seeking information and explanations, attempting to overdo for the child (for example, bringing lots of things for the crib), focusing on the past (things I could or should have done). Some may want to avoid the infant because it is a reminder of alcohol, drug use, or other neglect during pregnancy.

Feelings: Low self-esteem, culpability, unworthiness, self-pity, remorse

Underlying statements: "I'm being punished for something I did, thought, or said." "I didn't mean to do it." "I never should have had this child." "It's my fault that my child is suffering." "I should have listened to my doctor."

Interventions: Whether it is real or imagined guilt, parents can be helped by giving them the opportunity to explore their feelings. Do not gloss it over by saying, "You shouldn't feel guilty" or "You didn't mean it." Guilt is a part of letting go of the old dream and learning how to build a new one.

Listen closely and restate the "feeling" statements, encourage exploration of feelings, affirm their experience, and show them you understand. Permit parents to talk about their feelings of loss. Identify feelings other than guilt when you see them. With real guilt (such as that felt by a parent who is a drug user), you might need to say, "You must feel terrible." Guilt can become immobilizing. If parents are immobilized, you may need to focus on the effects of guilt on parenting (for example, the parents may be focusing on their own guilt rather than on parenting tasks).

You might ask, "How is your guilt serving the baby? We need to focus on what we can do for the baby now."

Depression

Certain things must be intact in our lives in order to feel good as human beings. Parents need to feel competent and capable. They need to feel worthy and valuable and at least somewhat in control of the events in their lives.

Depression is the opposite of these feelings. A premature birth places some parents in conditions that are likely to lead to depression. It is a rare parent who has not felt overwhelmed and discouraged during this time.

Signs and cues: Weak affect, little eye contact, very few words, an attitude that nothing matters, lack of energy, inability to wake up, loss of appetite, frequent crying, neglect of self

Feelings: Failure, despair, hopelessness, lack of power, loss of control, incompetence, fear for infant's life

Underlying statements: "I cannot cope with this." "I am totally discouraged and defeated." "What's the point?" "Why should I go on?" "I want to give up, but I know I can't."

Interventions: Explore what is beneath the surface by helping parents give words to what they are experiencing. Sit down with the parents. Say, "Tell me more about that," actively listen, and help them express their feelings of being in flux, confused, and in turmoil. Help them to make transitions into other emotional states. For example, point out even the small ways they are in control, and help them regard their baby positively. Experiences other than depression offer new definitions and possibilities. Reinforce parents' efforts to build new definitions and dreams for their lives.

Anger

Anger is a powerful emotion waiting to surface. Many NICU parents feel a free-floating anger that might rest on anyone—physicians, family, God. Many parents are waiting to explode, and it is important that they do—within limits. If parents find a mistake in their infant's care, their anger can become a "vacation" from the impotence with which they live. Anger is common among NICU parents, although it is not always expressed. Some parents report holding their anger for fear of the health professional's response to them or their infant.

Signs and cues: Stiff body, clenched hands and face, aggression, closed posture or openly accusing gestures, flushed face, flow of energy and strength, blaming, angry at self, mate, doctor, nurse, God, other parents, normal babies

Feelings: Abandoned, let down, "like a victim", out of control, "going crazy"

Underlying statements: "This is not fair." "It is not my fault." "Someone must be to blame." "Is the universe fair?" "How could this have happened to me?". "The world is unjust." "Life is unfair." "Someone else must be in control."

Interventions: Understand the anger that parents express, and develop skills to handle it. Do not withhold information, mislead them, or tell them an outright lie. Hear their anger. Allow them to be angry. Let their anger roll over you or past you; realize that you may not be the target and try to not take it personally. Make a listening statement, such as "You sound angry." Most people will not stay in anger long. Through listening you can help parents transition into another state. Do not back off or look away. Remain calm, reflective, and assertive. Stay with the facts—not the interpretation of the facts.

Jealousy

The baby that the parents had planned on taking home, the homecoming celebration, the congratulations and visits from friends and neighbors—these events have not happened. Instead, the baby is in the care of others. Some parents who experience this separation and loss of control feel jealous of the professionals who have charge of their infant's care in the intensive care nursery. Under the circumstances, the parents' feelings are understandable. NICU professionals must be attuned to these feelings. They must let parents know that they, the parents, are important to their infant. The infant belongs to the parents.

Signs and cues: Avoidance of professionals, insincere politeness, asking questions which have no answer, wanting to be alone with the infant, becoming competitive with nurses

Feelings: Left out, clumsy and incompetent, powerless, fear of failure

Underlying statements: "You have my baby." "You are in control and I ought to be." "I don't like this setup." "This place is foreign, cold and impersonal." "The doctors and nurses are smooth compared to me." "I should know more about my own baby." "The professionals do things I don't like. They are not gentle; they hurt my infant and treat babies like objects." "My baby knows the nurse better than she knows me."

Interventions: Share your knowledge with parents. Help them become partners in the child's care. Do not try to show them you know more than they do. Help them understand the things they can do for their baby. Studies have shown that babies can recognize their mother's voice even in the womb. Tell parents this, and encourage them to talk to their infant. Remind parents that they are their infant's most important allies.

Denial

Parents often deny in order not to experience other emotional states. At one level, all denial is a denial of feelings. It protects parents from having to face the implications of a core loss. Denial buys time and may be keeping hope alive. It is unconsciously structured so that the parents can ease themselves into other emotional states. Denial is safer and more comfortable than the turmoil and pain of other states. Because denial is used to ward off unwanted feelings, it may be difficult to work with parents in that state.

Ironically, professionals enjoy working with people in denial because they often give an air of confidence, seem able to handle difficult matters, and appear to be unafraid of the consequences. No amount of reality, difficult prognosis, or dangerous prospects will dissuade someone who is in denial.

Levels of denial may include some of the following:

Denial of fact. "There is not a problem, and I don't want to know if there is one. If I don't pay attention, then everything might be okay." This is not a lie, but a powerful wish that everything will be all right.

Denial of implications. The physician reports, "Your baby is very small and fragile. We are doing everything we can, but it appears that there might be neurological damage and the eyes might be impaired." The parent responds, "Everything will be fine. We aren't worried. Our other children were slow, but now they are doing just fine."

Denial of feelings. Denial is protection from the pain of a core loss. "My baby has cerebral palsy, but there is no sense dwelling on it. We must get on with our lives and live with it." At one level this is admirable, but it may keep parents out of touch with their feelings and the opportunity for emotional growth.

Signs and cues: Unrealistic expectations about the infant, refusing to listen to professionals' concerns. A false optimism.

Feelings: "Everything is fine. Nothing is wrong with my baby." Optimistic, upbeat, accepting.

Underlying statements: "I won't let anything happen." "This will pass and everything will be just fine." "I know things aren't right, but I cannot face it all right now." "I cannot give up the dream." "It's going to be OK."

Interventions: Be honest with the parent, but try never to push the consequences too hard. Present the facts as you know them, and avoid interpretations. Look carefully for signs of other states, and attempt to reflect those. Getting in touch with new feelings can be insightful.

If and when parents do work through their denial, usually they will begin to live with their anxiety over the loss and begin to feel and confront what has happened to them.

■ SUMMARY

Learning to cope and adapt to an at-risk birth take a long time, but however long it takes, the process is not static. Parents who have or acquire the skills to cope with personal loss normally become stronger through their grieving. Some become stronger where they have been wounded. Often parents become much clearer about their values and stronger in living their lives. They learn the importance of social supports and work harder on their relationships with family and friends (Ross, 1980).

NICU staff can assist parents in a number of ways. Look for changes in parents and be aware of the shifts in their emotional states. Acknowledge how they feel. Tell them, "You seem strong today" or "Today seems to be a low day for you." Enable parents to talk and share their feelings. It does not have to be a long conversation, but it is important that you hear them.

Staff can offer parents permission to own their feelings and the openness to talk about how they feel. Helpful statements include, "Other parents have told me how confused they were at first"; "I would probably be angry, too"; or "It's not unusual to feel some guilt about the baby's birth." If the going gets a little rough, ask if they would like to talk to someone else. If you think they need more help, pursue alternatives with them—family, friends, mental health professionals, and church groups. Help them contact an NICU parent support group.

Above all, realize that the grieving process takes time. Giving up dreams and building new ones is not easy. Although time is on their side, parents may not see it at the moment. Share stories about parents who are like them who have made it. Provide them with the names of parents whom they might talk with about their experiences.

Finally, NICU staff can let parents know they are in this together as a team to help meet their baby's short- and long-term needs (Edwards & Allen, 1988). Encourage them to be a partner. By doing so, staff will help parents to reach the point where they know they are going to make it. Staff members will have been a major support in the process of helping families to be survivors in a very difficult situation.

■ REFERENCES

Affleck, G., Tennen, H., Allen, D., & Rowe, J. (1986, April). *Rebuilding shattered assumptions after the birth of high risk infants: Parents' adaption to the secondary stresses of newborn intensive care.* Paper presented at the Biennial Meeting of the international Conference on Infant Studies, Los Angeles.

Affleck, G., Tennen, H., McGrade, B., & Katzan, S. (1985). Causal and control cognitions in parent coping with chronically ill children. *Journal of Social and Clinical Psychology, 3*, 369-379.

Affleck, G., Tennen, H., & Rowe, J. (1991). *Infants in crisis: How parents cope with newborn intensive care and its aftermath.* New York: Springer-Verlag.

Affleck, G., Tennen, H., Rowe, J., & Higgins, P. (1990). Mothers' remembrances on newborn intensive care: A predictive study. *Journal of Pediatric Psychology, 15,* 67–81.

Bailey, D. B., Jr., & Simeonsson, R. J. (1988). *Family assessment in early intervention.* Columbus: Merrill.

Benfield, D. G., Lieb, S. A., & Reuter, J. (1976). Grief response of parents after referral of the critically ill newborn to a regional center. New England *Journal of Medicine, 284,* 975–978.

Bogden, R., Brown, M., & Foster, S. (1982). Be honest but not cruel: Staff-patient communication on a neonatal unit. *Human Organization, 41,* 6–16.

Briggs, D. (1985). *The impact on the family of having a newborn baby hospitalized on a newborn intensive care unit.* Unpublished doctoral dissertation, Brandon University, Waltham, MA.

Cole, S. (1987). Parental grieving. In H. W. Taeusch & M. W. Yogman (Eds.), *Follow-up management of the high-risk infant* (pp. 307–314). Boston: Little, Brown.

Crnic, K., Greenberg, M., & Slough, N. (1986). Early stress and social support influences on mothers' and high risk infants' functioning in late infancy. *Infant Mental Health Journal, 7,* 19–33.

Edwards, K. A., & Allen, M. E. (1988). Nursing management of the human response to the premature birth experience. *Neonatal Network, 6,* 82–86.

Epps, S. (1993). Labeling effects of infant health and parent demographics on nurses' ratings of preterm infant behavior. *Infant Mental Health Journal, 14,* 182–191.

Gardner, S. C., & Merenstein, G. B. (1986). Perinatal grief and loss: An overview. *Neonatal Network, 4,* 7–15.

Goldberg, S., & Divito, B. A. (1983). *Born too soon.* New York: W.H. Freeman.

Goldberger, J. (1987). Infants on acute care hospital units: Issues in stimulation and intervention. In N. Gunzenhauser (Ed.), *Infant stimulation* (pp. 111–121). Skillman, NJ: Johnson & Johnson.

Gorski, P. A. (1991). Developmental intervention during neonatal hospitalization: Critiquing the state of the science. *Pediatric Clinics of North America, 38,* 1469–1479.

Griffin, T. (1990). Nurse barriers to parenting in the special care nursery. *Journal of Perinatal Neonatal Nursing, 5*(2), 56–67.

Hughes, M., McCollum, J., Sheftel, D., & Sanchez, G. (1994). How parents cope with the experience of neonatal intensive care. *Children's Health Care, 23,* 1–14.

Hummel, P. A., & Eastman, D. L. (1991). Do parents of preterm infants suffer from chronic sorrow? *Neonatal Network, 10,* 59–65.

Hynan, M. T. (1986). Emotional reactions to premature birth: Anticipating grief. *Special Care, 4,* 22–23.

Johnson, S. H. (1979). *High-risk parenting: Nursing assessments and strategies for the family at risk.* Philadelphia: J.B. Lippincott.

Johnson, S. H. (1983). *A review of what is known and consideration of appropriate preventative intervention.* New Brunswick, NJ: Johnson and Johnson.

Kubler-Ross, E. (1969). *On death and dying.* New York: Macmillan.

Lindemann, E. (1944). Symptomatology and management of acute grief. *American Journal of Psychiatry, 101,* 141–148.

Littman, B. (1979). The relationship between medical events and infant development. In T. Field (Ed.), *Infants born at risk: Behavior and development* (pp. 53–66). Jamaica, NY: Spectrum.

Lopez, C. J. (1983). Early Experiences of premature infants and their care providers. *Zero to Three, 4,* 7–11.

McCauley, B. B., & McCauley, J. E. (1987). Continuing care: Parent's retrospective. In H. W. Taeusch & M. W. Yogman (Eds.), *Follow-up management of the high-risk infant* (pp. 331–337). Boston: Little, Brown.

Mehren, E. (1991). *Born too soon.* New York: Doubleday.

Rosenthal, C. J., Marscall, V. W., MacPherson, A. J., & French, J. (1980). *Nurses, patients and families.* New York: Springer-Verlag.

Ross, G. (1980). Parental responses to infants in intensive care: The separation issue reevaluated. *Clinics in Perinatology, 7,* 47–60.

Sammons, W. H., & Lewis, J. M. (1985). *Premature babies: A different beginning.* St. Louis: C. V. Mosby.

Schiff, H. S. (1977). *The bereaved parent.* New York: Penguin Books.

Taylor, P. M., & Hall, B. L. (1979). Parents' usual emotional reactions and adjustments to full-term and pre-term infants. *Seminars in Perinatalogy, 3,* 73–89.

Whetsell, M. V., & Larrabee, M. J. (1988). Using guilt constructively in the NICU to affirm parental coping. *Neonatal Network, 6,* 21–27.

Wyly, M. V., & Allen, J. (1990). *Stress and coping in the neonatal intensive care unit.* Tucson, AZ: Communication Skill Builders.

■ CHAPTER 9
Family Interventions

I get by with a little help from my friends.
The Beatles

■ INTRODUCTION

For the most part neonatal intensive care nurseries have followed an infant-centered philosophy and approach, and infants' survival and medical well-being have been the dominant concerns of the field. As a consequence, great advances have taken place and knowledge about premature infants grows daily.

But important psychosocial issues have been slow in gaining the notice they deserve. Work with infants is typically more valued than parent interventions even in non-life-threatening situations. Although lifesaving acute care for infants is the foremost priority in the NICU, opportunities should not be lost to move forward with a family-centered focus that addresses both infant care and the psychosocial needs of the infant's caregivers (Gennaro, 1985).

Health professionals in the NICU need to develop a family-centered philosophy that includes working in partnership with families as well as caring for infants. It is important to identify both the infant's and the family's needs, stressors and appropriate interventions.

"I'm here for the babies, not for the parents" is not an acceptable philosophy. In too many instances, family members have been treated in a sink-or-swim manner and have come out of the NICU experience with bitterness. "It was the worst experience of my life" is a remark that tells professionals they need to do more for families.

Just as NICU professionals provide appropriate developmental interventions to reduce infant stress and promote effective coping strategies, so too can they facilitate family coping in the adjustment to the neonatal intensive care unit. Doing this is a key element in family-centered care. In the process, NICU professionals and families learn to work with one another and develop mutual trust and respect, which in turn heightens the probability for productive communication and family involvement so important to an infant's long term care.

Parent stress and family crises are very real events associated with the birth of a premature infant or an infant at risk for developmental disabilities. Family members often experience high levels of stress during their encounter with a neonatal intensive care nursery.

We learned previously (Chapter 8) that all parents do not grieve in the same way. Not surprisingly, studies have shown that 75% of the mothers and fathers of NICU infants employ quite different coping skills to manage their infant's hospitalization (Affleck, Tennen, & Rowe, 1991). Compared to fathers, mothers are more willing to express their emotions. Also, mothers have been found to use a combination of coping strategies. Most use social support and look for meaning in the experience of having an infant in the NICU. Fathers cope most often by looking for meaning in the NICU experience, followed by seeking social support (Affleck et al., 1991). Miles and Carter (1985) reported that parents use problem-solving coping strategies more often than emotion-focused coping to manage their intensive care experience.

Research on the impact of the intensive care nursery experience on families has shown that family coping strategies differed among families. Some families used daily coping, which included taking things one day at a time and appreciating the small victories in their childrens' lives (Able-Boone & Stevens, 1994a). The coping strategies used depended on the amount of caregiving needed for the child as well as the availability of social support networks (Able-Boone & Stevens, 1994b).

Some families have a very low tolerance for what is involved in a preterm birth crisis; others adapt quite easily and in between are a wide range of differences. Affleck and Tennen (1991) found that parents have substantial variation in their emotional reactions to their infant's hospitalization. It is important to remember that each family comes to the hospital with its own set of values, needs, attitudes, and wishes and that each of these elements influences how they cope with the experience.

NICU health providers and the families of NICU babies are made up of ordinary people serving in extraordinary circumstances. Having made this point, it is not contradictory to say that among NICU staff and families there are extraordinary people performing at a very high level. Today, important psychosocial changes that need to be made in NICUs are being made because neonatal staff and families articulate the needs and press for change (Harrison, 1993; Londner, 1993).

A poignant thing happened during the 1988 Winter Olympics. Dan Jansen, an American speed skater who was an early favorite for a medal, went into the competition knowing that his sister was dying of cancer. She died just before he skated his first event. In the competition, he fell on the first turn. In his second event, he took another spill. He had never fallen in either the trials or prior competitions. During the award ceremonies he was given the medal for "the athlete who overcame the most adversity." In accepting the medal he said, "I am very pleased to learn that there is a 'silver lining' in the midst of all this sorrow and sadness."

This theme very aptly and appropriately symbolizes the health professionals' task in regard to families in the NICU. Their task is to provide the knowledge, support, skills, and understanding that will enable parents to see the "silver lining" in the midst of their anxiety and concern for their infant. It should be noted, however, that family members usually do not experience the level of stress described for Dan Jansen, because most premature infants survive with a good chance for normal development.

This awareness of the extraordinary nature of the NICU, combined with the realization of the struggle in which many families are engaged, has led to an increasing chorus calling for a shift in paradigm. The focus has been shifting for over a decade, and many NICUs are becoming more family-centered in their care. It is by no means an even playing field. One can visit nurseries who fully welcome and engage the family and some who have only begun the journey to help families find the "silver lining."

This is a time of challenge and opportunity. NICU parents and professionals need to develop the partnership that will ensure progress toward a NICU paradigm wherein cooperation both enhances the long-term quality of vulnerable babies' lives and also serves infants' families.

In this chapter we will examine interventions that promote family support and involvement in the NICU. These include environmental interventions, grief interventions, psychosocial interventions, and communication interventions. Ways to involve family members in nonmedical aspects of infant care and in developmental care will be highlighted. Ways that NICU staff can provide continuity of care through discharge will be discussed. Developing the Individualized Family Service Plan (IFSP) for families with infants with disabilities will be reviewed.

■ PERSONAL CONTROL

A review of the parent experience in Chapter 8 will remind you that the NICU is a place where by definition persons other than the infant's parents are in charge of an infant's care. Consequently issues of control, perceptions of parenthood, and influencing outcomes are high on the agenda of the NICU culture. "Whose baby is it?" is a question on the minds of many parents.

The idea that we influence the events in our lives is important to our view of ourselves and to our self-esteem. When we lose control over events we feel helpless and incompetent (Thompson, 1985). The literature on stress and coping pays a great deal of attention to the issue of control. Perceived or real, control is central to how people handle themselves in threatening situations (Greenberg, 1987; Seligman, 1975; Taylor, 1986). In the view of many researchers, the absence of perceived control is viewed as a source of stress, of feeling overwhelmed, and seeing life as a struggle.

It has generally been assumed that individuals have better outcomes when they believe that they control the threatening experiences in their life. The NICU experience, however, raises some unique questions about this and the answers are not always as clear as one might assume. Ambiguities regarding this issue have been identified, and there appear to be circumstances in which people willingly give up control. Miller (1980) suggested that the health care setting may allow one to relinquish control because we assume that care providers are better equipped to handle the problem.

Parents in the NICU clearly differ over their level of involvement and need for control. While we know this from experience, recently researchers have identified some of the differences. Affleck et al. (1991) found that up to one half of NICU parents interviewed were quite willing to surrender the care of their infant to health professionals. This yielding to an "expert" they called **vicarious control**. Parents felt the demands were too complex and that they could not handle the tasks.

However, approximately 20% of the interviewed parents sought and received some degree of control in the care of their infant. This active participation and cooperation was identified as **participatory control**. The NICU care provider was viewed as in charge of the care and in turn provided information and opportunities for the parent to become involved in the decisions and care of the infant. This group of parents were rarely critical of staff.

Another group, approximately 20% of the subjects, were described as **conflicted**. They were unwilling to concede control to the staff but were unable to gain a comfortable level of participation in the NICU. Criticisms about communication, lack of information, a confusing and chaotic place, and an unwelcome feeling were common in this group.

These results underscore the importance of assessing families, not only regarding their marital status, cultural roots, socioeconomic level, and level of information receptivity, but also about their emotional state and level of inquiry and needs in relation to their infant. An improper assessment of the family, making incorrect assumptions about families, or not relating well with a parent can lead to very negative experiences among staff, parents, and others (Bogdan, Brown, & Foster, 1982; Griffin, 1990).

■ ENVIRONMENTAL INTERVENTIONS

The NICU environment has often been described as potentially stressful for high-risk infants (Jones, 1982; Stevens, 1981). Families, too, are likely to experience stress in this environment (Cohen, 1982; Perehudoff, 1990). The impact of an intensive care environment can compound the anxiety and grief of families and make coping difficult at best (Zeanah & Canger, 1983). But not all NICUs are equally stressful. Some units institute procedures to reduce environmental stress and to help parents while others pay little attention to the impact of their NICU on the family experience (Grobstein, 1982).

Londner (1993), a parent of a premature infant, described her reactions to a NICU in a presentation at a conference of neonatologists:

> To ordinary people like us, the NICU seemed like organized chaos. The lights were bright. The techno-noise of the monitors and other machinery were unnerving to an outsider.
>
> Then there was the music; the incessant noise of loud pop music. When we asked why there was music in our baby's nursery, music neither he nor we had requested, we were told it was to "keep the nurses up," to keep their spirits high.
>
> About a year later I heard a piece of music on the car radio and burst into tears without realizing why; then I recognized the song, the theme from "Hill Street Blues," as one of the tunes blaring endlessly in the NICU while Michael was there. (Londner, 1993, p. 12)

Too often a neonatal intensive care unit is noisy and intense. On their first visit to see their infant in the NICU, family members may be unable to attend to their infant because they are so overwhelmed with the noise, crowd of nurses, physicians and support personnel, machinery, and relentless medical procedures. In addition, parents may be shocked by their infant's physical appearance. It is not surprising that many parents have been frightened by the NICU environment (Ensher & Clark, 1986; Miles, Funk, & Kasper, 1992).

To make matters worse, sometimes no effort is made to orient families to the nursery when they enter a NICU; some parents are tentatively looking for their baby while being ignored by NICU staff.

They feel out of place and unwelcome in the unit. This only intensifies whatever feelings of incompetence and helplessness they may already have.

> "We're here to see our daughter," he said. " Emily Butterfield." "Butterfield?" the nurse repeated. "Butterfield?" "Look, I was just up here an hour or so ago," Fox said. "She was born this morning. She's in the intensive care area." "Butterfield?" the nurse said again, but buzzed us in anyway.
>
> The receptionist's desk was still empty. There was no one around to instruct us in K9 rules and regulations. "You'll need to wear gowns," the nurse said over her shoulder as she headed down the hallway. Without looking at us, she pointed at a small room a few feet from the reception area. "You can get them in there." (Mehren, 1991, pp. 56–57)

Family members often have little or no privacy with their infant. This is particularly distressing when the infant is critically ill or dying. In some nurseries there is no comfortable place for parents to sit with their baby. A mother's first attempt to breast feed her infant is likely to be quite public, and consultations with physicians or nurses may take place in full view of the rest of the nursery. Recently, a neonatal nurse recounted seeing a physician delivering bad news to a mother about her infant's prognosis. The mother was alone and crying, leaning against the wall of the hallway leading to the unit. While the physician talked, staff and parents walked around them. Such insensitivities only heighten parents' feelings of sorrow and alienation. Equally important, these experiences are long remembered.

NICU staff can make environmental interventions that are useful and supportive for families. Many environmental interventions designed to reduce infant stress also can help family members in their coping efforts. Environmental interventions that are likely to help family members include these:

- Lower the lights when possible.
- Reduce noise levels, for example, talk quietly, respond to monitor alarms, eliminate loudspeakers, muffle telephone bells.
- Conduct rounds discussions away from infants' isolettes.
- Turn off the radio.
- Speak quietly to family members and encourage a restful atmosphere during their visit.
- Ask what parents need to be comfortable. If at all possible respond to their requests.
- Provide a comfortable rocking chair or seat for use by family members.
- Minimize activities that might be distracting during family visits.

■ If family members visit during a particularly busy time suggest a less busy time to visit.

■ Whenever possible, provide privacy for families visiting their infant. A movable folding screen or curtain will provide privacy. If these are not available, position family members to face the infant rather than out toward the open nursery room.

■ Designate a small room for "alone" time for parents and intact infants. Such small rooms can also be used as breast feeding rooms, overnight rooms for parents and infant prior to discharge, as well as for families whose infants are dying or have died.

■ Identify a private place for consultation with parents.

■ Organize quiet time in the unit. Encourage parents to use that time to sit quietly with their infant.

■ Provide a quiet, pleasant, smoke-free waiting room for families. If possible place childrens' chairs and a table with picture books and games in the room. Place notebooks in which parents can paste pictures and write notes about their experiences in the NICU and about their special memories and thanks.

■ Place a bulletin board in the family waiting room or above the scrub sink where parents can post letters or photos from or about NICU graduates.

■ Provide a light refreshment area for family members.

■ PSYCHOSOCIAL INTERVENTIONS

NICU health professionals can use a variety of psychosocial interventions to help family members move from feeling anxious and inadequate to feeling secure and competent. To do this, health professionals do not have to become psychologists or social workers, rather they should work to increase their sensitivity to and support for family needs (Bass, 1991). Once they are sensitive to family needs, health professionals need to become successful at implementing appropriate interventions that benefit both infants and families. Although psychosocial interventions should take place throughout the infant's hospitalization, they begin when the family first visits the NICU.

The First Visit to the Nursery

The family's first visit to the nursery is critical and can be traumatic (Edwards & Allen, 1988). Their impressions, feelings, and experiences on that first visit play a key role in parenting and determining later parent-infant interactions (Gennaro, 1991; Goldberg & DiVitto, 1983; Harrison, 1990) (see Figure 9–1).

Mehren (1991) described her experience as a new parent of a premature infant:

> Fox and I had just had a baby, a normal event. But in the process, all three of us had been catapulted into an odd and unknown universe where the natives spoke their own language, a tongue called Acronymic. They had their own strange customs and their own quaint costumes. Medicine was the prevailing form of government: What the textbooks taught was the law of the land. Science and technology were the religion here, and the doctors were the keepers of the temple, that much was absolutely clear. The rules were based equally on luck and uncertainty. (Mehren, 1991, p. 46)

Things that can be done to make that first family visit less stressful include:

- Arrange for someone to meet the family at the nurserywaiting room and provide a brief orientation to the unit. "Veteran parents", or a social worker, a receptionist, or a nurse might be identified as the greeter.
- Have the NICU nurse caring for the baby be available if possible to greet the parents as they enter the nursery. Parents should be seated by the isolette so that they can see their baby.
- Provide explanations about the infant's appearance or medical condition but keep explanations brief and free of medical jargon. Read and assess parent cues and coping skills.
- Have a NICU health professional available to answer parents' questions. If a medical procedure must be done during their visit, explain the purpose of the procedure simply and clearly.
- Reduce unnecessary distractions. Listen to the parents attentively.
- Allow family members space and privacy.
- Encourage parents/family members to visit often. If daily visits are not possible, arrange a daily calling time.
- Provide pamphlets and other written material which describe the NICU and give parents information about premature infants.

During their initial visit to the NICU some families may be told that their infant has a potentially disabling or life-threatening condition. Often it is the attending neonatologist who breaks the news. This is a difficult situation, but parents who have had this experience

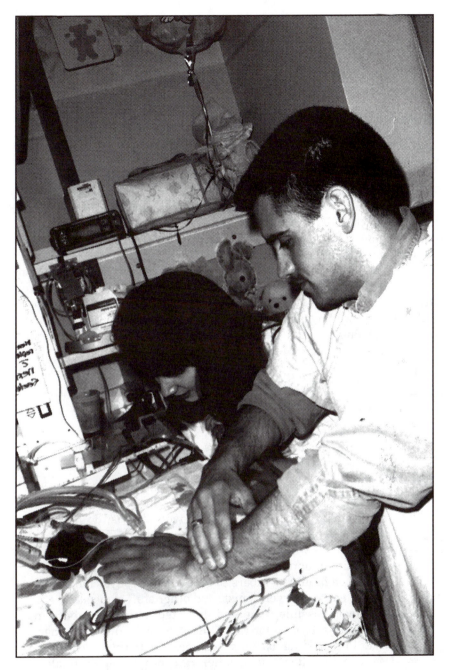

FIGURE 9–1. A family visits with their infant. (Photograph courtesy of Children's Hospital of Buffalo Department of Medical Photography.)

recommend that the information be presented in an honest, straightforward, yet compassionate manner. It is important that the person who presents the diagnoses is sensitive to feelings and conveys a caring attitude (Bogdon et al., 1982).

Ongoing Hospitalization

While research shows that both parents are distressed by the birth and hospitalization of a preterm infant, mothers report more distress than fathers (Affleck et al., 1991; Levy-Schiff, Sharir, & Mogilner, 1987). Over time, the uncertainty and anxiety of family members lessen (Miles et al., 1992). Individual family members, however, will respond to the NICU experience based on their own cultural values, their coping skills, their infant's condition, and the support they receive from staff and others in their lives.

NICU staff need to evaluate each families' responses at admission to determine appropriate interventions. Because neonatal health professionals are central mediators in interventions with families and their infants, they need to have a range of alternative interventions available for use with families. They can start the process of selecting appropriate interventions by asking themselves the following questions:

- What does this family need?
- What are appropriate interventions to use with the various family members?
- Which of these interventions is likely to help most?

Some psychosocial interventions that NICU professionals can use to assist parents during their infant's hospitalization are:

- Collaborate rather than compete with parents. For example, avoid statements that place parents in competition with professionals as the infant's caregiver, that is, do not verbally or nonverbally act as if it is your baby.
- Identify times when concerns and questions can be addressed without interruptions. Do this in a private, quiet place.
- Encourage family members to talk with the physician, social worker, early interventionist, and other staff as needed.
- Whenever possible, involve interested family members in caregiving activities for their infant, that is, diaper change, swaddling, nesting, bathing, temperature taking.
- Use a small yellow flag or other agreed upon signal to alert NICU staff that there is a very sick or dying baby.
- Support extended family visits.

- Acknowledge parent discomfort, for example, "I know this must be difficult;" "This can be a difficult place."
- Help parents identify their infant's unique characteristics. Point out the infant's behaviors or milestones. Inform them of their infant's daily routines, for example, how long the infant sleeps and when the infant feeds.
- Identify social support links for families.
- Respect cultural differences in family members' approach to their infant.
- Provide information on a regular basis. Use simple, direct language. Identify resource material when appropriate.
- Encourage family members to talk with other parents or become involved in parent-to-parent support. Respect their decision not to share their experience with others.
- Provide support in family decision making around procedures or ethical issues involving their infant.

■ COMMUNICATION INTERVENTIONS

Families are a complex dynamic system that has been likened to a hanging mobile; if one of the links is taken or broken, the mobile (or a family) is thrown out of balance. The NICU experience places a family's balance in jeopardy. NICU professionals not only must place themselves in parents' shoes, but also should be ready to communicate effectively with parents. Effective communication begins with the desire to understand and empathize with the other person. Communication can be a major source of stress in people's lives. Although what we say is very important, particularly in the context of the NICU experience, the way we say it may be much more important (Sammons & Lewis, 1985). This chapter will give you an opportunity to examine your communication style and perhaps identify some ways you can communicate better with parents.

All communication is a transaction between two or more persons. These transactions can be viewed as either negative or positive, stressful or relaxing, rewarding, or unpleasant. Positive interactions create relative ease, whereas negative exchanges tend to cause conflict and stress. Although most people want to make their transactions a positive experience, this goal cannot be achieved all the time. Nonetheless, every effort should be made to keep communication at a low stress level (Verderber & Verderber, 1995).

Generally speaking, most people seek positive experiences and try to avoid negative ones. If communication causes high stress and people have a choice, they will not want to repeat it. On the other hand if communication creates little stress or is rewarding for others, people are more likely to repeat those transactions.

Communication is a very important area to examine in attempting to reduce unnecessary stress in the NICU (Schmerber, 1982). Although most individuals view themselves as good communicators, a close look at the reactions of others can reveal communication patterns that need improvement.

A variety of communication styles may be used depending on the context. Each style comes with its own set of verbal and nonverbal messages which mirror the speaker's values, feelings of self-worth, and regard for other persons.

When you speak with another person, all of you speaks. This person has at least three levels. There are the **words** you use, your **body language** (including facial expression, position and posture, breathing, and voice tone) and the **feelings** you have at the time. Your words may say one thing while your body position expresses a contrary feeling. For example, what is being said when a nurse greets parents with, "Hello! How are you? Good to see you!" but immediately turns her back or stays far away from the parents for the rest of their visit with their infant? What is really being said by a health professional who leans into a nursery doorway fifteen feet from the parents and loudly carries on a one-way conversation with the parents about breast feeding? In both instances, the health care provider's body actions let the parents know that they really don't want to communicate or are too busy to communicate.

A person's communication style is learned in childhood and is "perfected" over the years. It is difficult to totally change a communication style, and often that is not a desirable goal. However, if you want to modify some negative elements of your communication style, you should try the following:

■ Understand the impact, positive and negative, that your present style has upon other people.

■ Begin to make choices about the style you use presently in various contexts. Understand the impact you are having upon parents then choose how you will act. People can be passive in some situations and more aggressive in others. You may choose to continue deferring to others' wishes or to continue with a style that makes parents feel uncomfortable. The point is, whatever you do be aware of what you are doing and of your impact on others. Do not be unthinking. Make choices about what you do.

■   Identify new skills that will modify your present style. Generally, the most effective communication style is the assertive style, and new skills should probably come from the assertive communication model, which is discussed below.

Assertive communication is direct and concrete (Bower & Bower, 1991). Specific statements or direct questions about information, thoughts, needs, and feelings are made. When using assertive communication, you have regard for the rights and feelings of others as well as for yourself. Before jumping in with information, the speaker assesses the emotional state of the other person. Questions are answered in clear language. When assertive communication is used with parents in the NICU, they will feel that they are being regarded.

Assertiveness does not mean that the speaker takes a lot of "air time," for example, talking too much or not allowing others to speak. Rather, an assertive communicator listens attentively and actively to let people know they have been heard. Assertive communicators will be comfortable with appropriate silences even when they are prolonged. They will make direct requests and refusals without apology. They will give and receive compliments comfortably.

They negotiate and compromise without sacrificing principles. They are comfortable starting and stopping conversations involving small talk or important parenting issues. They accept feedback and can be questioned without becoming defensive.

Assertive speakers are physically near the person with whom they speak. They convey openness, interest, and a readiness to listen. They have an air of quiet strength and self-assurance. They are relaxed and erect. They make good eye contact and speak in a calm, relaxed, firm manner.

An assertive style combined with empathetic listening is the most effective means of achieving the best results between two parties. It is the means by which all persons' needs are most likely to be heard and addressed.

Here are some examples of assertive communication:

"Mrs. Jones, you told me you would call the nursery at 1:00 P.M., but you didn't call until 5:00 P.M. when I was doing vital signs. I would appreciate your calls during times that are convenient for both you and me. If 1:00 P.M. is not convenient, maybe we need to agree on another time."

"I appreciate your regular visits to the NICU, Mr. McNamara."

"Nurse Smith, the radio in the nursery is disturbing infant Cane's sleep. It would be better for him if you turned it low. Thank you."

Barriers to Communication

There is considerable evidence that NICU staff members truly want to communicate with parents (Gorski, 1987). Care providers regularly seek out parents to talk; they provide information on a regular basis, telephone parents at critical junctures and invite parents to call any time. Many nurseries have an open visitation policy and encourage parents to interact with their infants.

Despite these and other positive activities, observers note that, with exceptions, NICU care providers and particularly physicians, spend relatively little time communicating with parents. If we accept the goals of family-centered care which include empowering families, enhancing parenting skills, assisting the attachment process, and facilitating parents' knowledge and understanding of their infant, we need to ask ourselves what prevents us from communicating more with parents.

Some visitors to a critical care nursery have said they feel like they have entered a landed spacecraft. This high-technology environment is crowded with incubators, ventilators, oxygen hoods, and much other equipment essential for the infants' survival. This very busy community, with its tiny developing premature infants, small fragile infants, and large infants with medical problems is a very busy place that does not provide easy access to parents. Indeed, it is often a difficult for parents to even establish personal contact with their infant who is hooked up to monitors and busy with care providers.

The lack of privacy, feeling inadequate and overwhelmed, uncertain about parenting, fearing attachment to an infant who is at risk, and experiencing an emotional roller coaster are only some of the psychological problems parents experience in the NICU. The parent perspective is primarily social/emotional and is sometimes difficult for the health professional to grasp. Nonetheless, identifying the psychosocial needs of parents in the NICU is just as important as identifying infant needs (Bogden et al., 1982).

This leads us to consider still another barrier to good communication, the attitude and perspective health care providers bring to their relationship with parents. In our 10 years of working with NICU staff, we have identified a host of attitude barriers that are raised by health care providers and parents. They include:

- Becoming overly attached to an infant patient; viewing the patient as "my baby"
- Being very territorial and thinking your space or role is being infringed upon

- Believing that care provider skills belong only to the professional
- Believing that staff does caregiving and parents do parenting
- Seeing parent involvement as an infringement upon professional demands
- Viewing parents as less capable than nurses or NICU health providers
- Envying parents who get to hold and love the child, leaving the nurse with the less emotionally satisfying aspects of care
- Approaching parents with suspicion. Thinking that parents are not allies but there to scrutinize the surrogate caregiver
- Seeing families as a source of stress and frustration
- Believing that teaching skills to parents is unimportant and takes too much time
- Taking the position that I am here for medical intervention only
- Thinking that I can work with good families but not with parents I do not value, for example, parents whose economic status, lifestyle, background, language, and culture are different from mine.

In summary, families have psychosocial needs and there are obstacles to meeting those needs. But when good contact is established with parents, they are empowered in their role as the infants' caregiver (Oster, 1984). Becoming aware of obstacles that stand in the way of developing a positive and cooperative relationship; can be the first step in becoming better communicators and enablers of parent functions in the NICU.

Listening Skills

Listening is critical to good communication. Parents in the NICU who feel that the staff listens to them feel less stress and frustration (Barnard, Snyder, & Spietz, 1984).

Paul Simon's lyrics in "Sounds of Silence" aptly describe what substitutes for listening in many of our relationships.

And in the naked light I saw . . .
People talking without speaking,
People hearing without listening,
People writing songs that voices never shared . . .

It is important to listen to one another and to know that messages are being shared. By actively listening, NICU health professionals can share messages with parents. These are steps you can follow:

1. Get ready. Check parents' emotional state and their readiness to communicate. Are they ready to speak, to listen, or to be quiet? Check yourself and your readiness to listen. Should you begin right away, finish what you are doing, or wait until you are ready?

2. Listen actively. Focus your attention totally on the other person. Shut out distractions as much as possible. Ask for clarification of thoughts and feelings ("I'm not sure I understand"; "I'm not clear about what is upsetting you"; "Do you want to tell me more?"; "Can you be more specific about that?"). Keep the channels open until the person has been heard.

3. Provide confirmation. Let parents know you heard their thoughts and their feelings ("It sounds like you are being bombarded by so many people right now"; "I understand you are getting conflicting messages from the staff"; "I see you are feeling exhausted from running around." Share some of your feelings. "I'm upset that you aren't getting more help from your family. You have every right to be angry about that"). Don't be afraid to share some of your own feelings when it is appropriate.

Delay Statements

In certain situations it is important not to continue the communication. Conflicts might be developing, criticisms are being leveled, or one of the communicators is becoming too passive or too aggressive. The communicators may need to take a break. Delays can give you time to do several things:

1. to understand what is going on with the other person. What is that person feeling?
2. to understand what is going on with you.
3. to analyze what is being said.
4. to figure out how to get back on track.

Statements to use when a delay might help include these:

"We seem to have drifted from our subject. Maybe we need a break and then get back to ..."

"Let's slow down. This is too important to rush through."

"I think I've been doing all the talking."

"That's a good point. Let me think about that for a while."

"I must be getting tired. Can we take a break?"

"Can you state that differently? I'm not sure I understand."

"We're getting upset. It's such a sensitive issue."

"I know this is important to you. Can I have a little time to think about it?"

"You (or I) appear to be getting upset. Could we take a short break?"

"I don't want you to feel pressured. Let's talk about this the next time we get together."

"We've covered a lot of ground. We may need some time to think it all over."

These can be very useful breaks that enable speakers to return to assertive communication.

■ GRIEF INTERVENTIONS

Grief is a painful process, and acute grief is debilitating and immobilizing. Because parents of preterm infants may have intense feelings of grief and sadness (Taylor & Hall, 1979). NICU staff should be ready to give parents all the help they need (Bogdan et al., 1982; Haut, Peddicord, & O'Brien, 1994).

Start by watching the parents closely. Look for behavioral changes in parents that signal transition in emotional states. Over time you will see parents go through a wide range of states and responses very much like changeable weather. Many parents say their experience in the NICU is like being on a roller coaster. Feeling like you are "going crazy" while in grief is common.

To appropriately respond to parents NICU health professionals need to recognize and understand parent emotional states. They should not be surprised by rapid shifts in states or by the confusions that parents experience. In addition to providing support and empathy, health professionals should consider using these coping interventions:

1. **Help parents contain the impact of the loss**. A primary loss threatens a person's entire life and often is generalized to mean that "everything" is lost, ruined, and futile. NICU health providers can help parents make an

accurate assessment of what is lost, what is salvageable, and what aspects of their lives are still intact.

Placing a major loss in perspective is a delicate task. If a newborn has died, for example, never say, "Well, at least you have each other" or "At least your other children are healthy." Never minimize the loss, but attempt to help the parents understand that other parts of their lives are intact and need to be kept as stable as possible under the conditions. You can do this by discussing with them their areas of family stability. For example, you might say, "Yes, Amy is in fragile condition and we are all working to get her better. I know this must be a difficult time. Perhaps having your parents and husband to talk with will help you through this." Social support is very important to these families.

2. **Help parents understand the "normality" of grief**. Often a primary loss will make parents feel they are outside "normal society." Parents often will feel insecure when they grieve, even though loss is a common human experience. You can help by identifying feelings that parents in the NICU often have: shock, sadness, guilt. Point out that these feelings are not unusual; they are normal and expected. Make available first hand accounts of grief reactions written by parents of premature infants and link parents to other parents in NICU support groups so they can talk about their feelings if they wish.

3. **Enlarge the scope of parents' values**. People often define their lives in narrow ways that do not allow for the unexpected. An experience with loss often calls their value system into question. Parents may need assistance in understanding the need to broaden their values to include living with things as they are now. They may feel that "Things like this don't happen to good people who try to play it by the rules." Parents need to accept that bad things can happen to good people.

Experiencing a premature birth alters a family's life in many unanticipated ways. You can help family members redefine their lives by helping them cope with changes they had not planned for (Miles & Carter, 1985). Help them identify manageable tasks related to their infant's hospitalization—tasks such as a daily visit or daily phone call to the nursery, or setting up a consultation with the attending physician. Have them bring something in for the baby. Help them focus on the present situation with the infant rather than on the future. To help reduce negative feelings about the experience, point out their baby's behaviors and competencies. Show parents what they can do to interact with their baby. Listen attentively when parents ask, "Why did this have to happen?" Inform them that there are no clear answers to the "whys" of premature births. It may be useful to provide several examples of other parents who followed all the guidelines during pregnancy and still had a premature birth.

4. **Focus on attachments and assets**. During a crisis or primary loss, most of us realize that our real assets are not material things but rather our attachments, our family, and friends. Families in the crisis of a preterm birth have an opportunity to come closer together. NICU staff members can help them to understand the need for greater intimacy, closeness, and mutual support in this situation.

   Families can be assisted by affirming their attachments with one another and by focusing on the important things they have. If possible, involve family members in collaborating with you in caregiving activities. Many nurseries encourage visits by grandparents and siblings. Suggest ways that family members can support one another. Refer them to other families who have been through the experience.

5. **Integrate the loss**. Parents do not have to view themselves as victims. Even sorrow can be integrated and transformed into learning about ourselves and about life. In his book, *Man's Search for Meaning*, Frankl (1963) described his experiences in a concentration camp. He stated that everything important can be taken away from us, including our dignity, but still we have the power to choose what attitude we take toward what has happened to us. Our attitude will help us to move beyond the question, "Why did this happen to me?" and ask instead, "Now that this has happened, what is my best course of action?" NICU families must decide how and in what way they are going to experience their loss and learn from it.

   Listen to parents discuss various courses of action. Point out that they do have choices, even if they are small ones. Acknowledge that it is a difficult situation but their approach toward it is their own choice. Provide them with examples of parents who coped well in the face of similar crisis, for example, an adolescent mother who asked family members to accompany her when she visited the nursery.

Whenever possible, encourage parents to talk with other parents who have been through the experience. Hearing how other parents have coped can be enormously helpful to parents, particularly in the early stages of their infant's hospitalization.

There are some parents, however, who do not want to share their experience with others. Respect their decision. Gender, race, education, cultural background, or socio-economic class could affect the way we communicate with people we do not know. Any one or combination of these factors could account for differences in open or closed communication. Be sensitive to the differences and alert to the needs of the variety of parents.

In the early stages of a family's grief, NICU health professionals are in a position to help them begin to cope and to understand their feelings of loss. Support, realistic optimism, and devotion and concern for the baby will help families in this process.

Before we leave this section on assisting families in grief, let us also condsider the NICU staff and their need to grieve. The staff, like parents, are ordinary people who happen to work in an extraordinary setting. In this setting, staff see a whole range of infants from the viable to very sick and dying infants. Staff are involved and often become attached to their fagile patients. The death of an infant is an ever present reality in Level 3 NICUs. Staff who work with these patients are often faced with the experience of grief over their loss. In our work with over 400 NICU staff throughout the country, staff members regularly cite caring for very ill infants and infant death as major stressors. Several studies have confirmed our observations (Benica, Longo, & Barnsteiner, 1992; Vachon & Parkes, 1985).

Research studies indicate that death in the NICU leaves staff feeling helpless and sad (Downey, Bengiamin, Hever, & Juhl, 1995). All of the research and personal testimony point to the need to grieve and share feelings with others.

Support in this coping process comes from a variety of sources, including co-workers for reassurance that staff members did all they could, support from "those who have been there," and talking with the infant's family and one's own family and friends. A common source of staff support is talking with a chaplain or psychologist. Staff can also gain comfort from attending the infant's funeral services. Meditation and excercise can help, crying is important to many, while some staff prefer being alone or taking time out.

In the past few years, NICUs have acknowledged the need for fostering formal and informal discussions on grief. Some NICUs have established bereavement teams to assist staff and family members.

Many NICUS encourage continued staff education to improve listening and support skills related to bereavement (Downey et al., 1995).

FAMILY INVOLVEMENT IN DEVELOPMENTAL CARE INTERVENTIONS

Neonatal health professionals play a key role in facilitating family participation in their infant's developmental care. This important process promotes positive relations between parents and their infant and also more positive long-term consequences for the infant.

Currently researchers are concerned that high-risk preterm infants are over represented in reported developmental disabilities and infant and child abuse (Gilkerson, Gorski, & Panitz, 1990). This is not surprising since the physical qualities and behavioral patterns of these infants often have a negative impact on families (Hertzig & Mittleman, 1984; Miles, Funk, & Kasper, 1991). Compared to full-term infants, young preterm infants are more irritable, look away more often in social exchanges, and are generally far less socially responsive to their caregivers. And caregivers often respond to their fragile, often unattractive and unresponsive infants by feeling tense and anxious, which may have a negative impact on subsequent interactions (Trause & Kramer, 1983).

Involving families early on in the developmental care of their premature infant can greatly assist the attachment process between parent and infant (see Figure 9–2) and consequently reduce family stress (Hughes, McCollum, Sheffel, & Sanchez, 1994) and enhance parental self-confidence (Flynn & McCollum, 1989). Suggested interventions include these:

- Point out the infant's unique behaviors and competencies. Ask parents or family members to identify any special characteristics they observe in their infant.
- Help parents recognize their infant's special interaction signals and suggest appropriate responses.
- Help parents distinguish between their infant's "time-out" signals of stimulus overload and their self-comforting behaviors. Support developmental interventions that match the signals. Help parents recognize when the infant is too fragile to tolerate any simulation. Guide parents, if necessary, in promoting their infant's self-comforting behaviors such as hand-to-mouth maneuvers, foot clasping, flexion, and midline positioning.
- Outline the infant's expected course of development. Help parents reconcile their expectations for the infant's development with the reality of the infant's likely development.

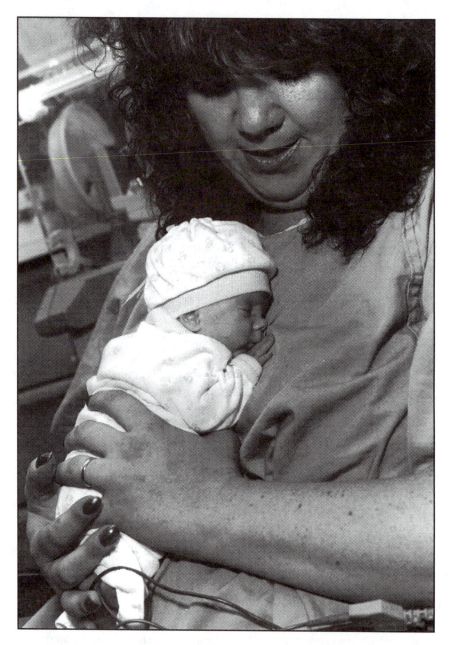

FIGURE 9–2. A preterm infant is cuddled by her mother. (Photograph courtesy of Children's Hospital of Buffalo Department of Medical Photography.)

- As soon as possible encourage parents to change diapers and to lift the baby to remove the diaper pad. When possible have parents assist in temperature taking, bathing, and feeding their infant.
- Watch the baby with the parents. Point out changes in behavioral states. Discuss appropriate interventions to use when the baby is alert and can tolerate stimulation. Then try the interventions.
- Help parents position their baby in supine, prone and side-lying position when appropriate. Show them how to use blanket rolls for containment. Demonstrate ways to handle and move their infant gently and slowly.
- When parents are holding or looking at their infant, position them so that they can receive positive feedback from the infant. Identify the infant's responses to parents' appropriate interactions as a way to let parents know that they are effective caregivers.
- As the infant matures, plan developmentally appropriate activities with the parent that match the infant's tolerance and capabilities.
- Involve parents in designing a developmental care plan for their infant.

When they involve parents and family members in the non-medical aspects of their infant's developmental care, NICU health professionals are including parents as partners in serving their infant (Plaas, 1994). Professionals should view their role as both facilitators and teachers in this important process, and some family members will take more time than others. In any event the desired outcomes are clear. The infant benefits while parents experience control in the NICU environment and gain confidence as parents.

■ TRANSITION INTERVENTIONS

For families of premature infants, the transition from hospital to home is a long anticipated event. For many parents it represents a step toward the normal birth experience they never had. For some families, the excitement of the homecoming follows a long period of hospitalization in which they often experienced anxiety and stress. Despite this, among family members the transition to home can evoke fears and doubts about their ability to care for their infant on their own (Salitross, 1986). While the infant is in the NICU, the NICU staff bear the major responsibility for the infant's care. Family members usually participate in some but not all of the nonmedical caregiving activities and are usually supported in important decision making by NICU medical staff. Upon discharge, the care responsibilities shift dramatically to the family.

> As we left the nursery, I kept looking back. Ray noticed my continued glance at the NICU as we waited for the elevator. My heart was pounding as he asked what was the matter. I told him I felt like we were kidnapping Josh and he wasn't ours to keep. I just knew any minute somebody was going to come running down the hallway yelling "Come back with that baby." It seemed to take the elevator forever to get us to the lobby. Once we got into the sun and the warm August air hit my face, I knew we were free. He was ours and we were going to care for him from now on. (Steichen, 1992, personal communication)

NICU health professionals tend to view discharge as the successful end to hospitalization. But families often view discharge differently. For many of them discharge will in fact be the beginning of a long process that involves ongoing medical and therapy services, seeking early intervention services and linking to community support (Bruder & Walker, 1990; Sabbeth, 1984).

Current sophisticated medicine and technology not only keep 23- to 25-week gestational age infants alive, they also shorten hospital stays. In the process these same lifesaving measures also create developmental problems among very low birthweight infants. These needs must be addressed on a continual basis (Sheikh, O'Brien, & McCluskey-Fawcett, 1993). In some cases technology goes home with infants with complex medical problems. This means that health care continues in the home (Arenson, 1988).

Even when infants go home with no medical or developmental problems, parents may be unprepared to care for a premature baby (Hanline & Deppe, 1990). Premature infants are less active, less responsive, and more difficult to care for than are full-term infants. They often have feeding difficulties characterized by spitting up and slow food intake. Compared to full-term infants, premature infants have higher-pitched cries (Frodi et al., 1978). Unless parents are prepared to expect and manage these behaviors, they may doubt their abilities as competent caregivers (Bruder & Cole, 1991).

Sheikh et al. (1993) examined the quality of preparation parents receive for the NICU-to-home transition from the point of view of the parents and of NICU nurses. Following discharge, staff nurses and parents were asked to rate 44 topics on infant care and prematurity that could be included in discharge teaching. Parents and staff rated the importance of the topic for parents. Staff nurses and parents generally agreed on the nature of the information that should be included in preparing for discharge home. Topics included feeding, taking care of baby's health, and monitoring baby's health. Staff nurses agreed that most of the items were important to include and that information on them had been provided to parents. Parents, on the other hand, did not remember receiving much of the information. In fact, fewer than 50% of the parents remembered being instructed on general signs of illness, whereas only 38% recalled receiving information about infant growth and development. Although 94% of the nurses surveyed said parents were instructed about what to do if their babies were not eating enough, only 24% of parents recalled hearing that information. There were also large discrepancies in items such as "What to do when baby cries," "How to encourage baby to interact with mother," "Awareness of normal and delayed growth and development," and "Suggestions on ways to encourage baby's growth and development." The results of this study indicated that effective discharge teaching must be a high priority for NICUs and that teaching must utilize techniques that ensure that parents really learn the information.

Preparation for discharge from the NICU to home can provide a smooth transition for families who have healthy preterm infants or infants with complex medical needs (Arenson, 1988; Bruder & Walker, 1990). Families report that successful discharge from the intensive care setting to the home comes from careful planning that begins long before the actual discharge (Able-Boone & Stevens, 1994a, 1994b; O'Hare & Terry, 1988). Parents who are well informed, are skilled in caring for their infant and who have been fully integrated into the NICU, are better prepared for the transition home (McCluskey-Fawcett, O'Brien, Robinson, & Asay, 1992).

What does all of this mean for transition and discharge interventions? Recent data on successful transition from the NICU identify a number of critical elements (Flynn & McCollum, 1989; Hanline & Deppe, 1990; Pearl, Brown, & Myers, 1990).

■ A professional should be assigned to each family at the time of their infant's hospitalization. The professional's primary task is to provide families with information while their infant is in the hospital, to coordinate follow-up services after discharge and to facilitate any technical assistance that families might need. Some NICUs employ parents in this role.

■ A transition plan should be developed for each family. The plan should contain goals and objectives designed to meet the needs of individual families while in the NICU, in the transition period and at home. The plan should be developed with input from family members, NICU care providers, the transition professional and a community transition professional. Should the infant require early intervention services, the transition plan should be incorporated into the Individualized Family Service Plan (IFSP) specified by Part H of Public Law 99-457 (Krehbiel, Munsick-Bruno, & Lowe, 1991).

■ Case management for preterm infants with disabilities should begin in the NICU. The Individuals with Disabilities Education Act (IDEA:Public Law 99-457) extended the age range of free public education for persons with disabilities to include children from birth to five years. Public Law 99-457 mandates case managers to help the child and child's family receive the services provided by the state's early intervention program.

■ A community resource professional, such as a social worker or area resource coordinator should be identified while the family is in the NICU. This individual would help families, who require follow-up or early intervention programs, locate comprehensive community based intervention services and facilitate the family's transition to those services. In some NICUs an early interventionist is on staff and works with the transition professional and family to facilitate continuity of care.

■ Parent education should take place throughout their child's hospitalization, not just at the time of discharge. And it should not rely on lectures. Instead, parent education should use adult learning techniques that foster active learning. Parent education should focus on the needs of individual families (and family members) and include information on infant cues and behaviors, on infant care and development as well as medical care, monitoring the baby's health, practical aspects of parenting an infant, and information about prematurity. Information and skills should be at the educational level of the families and be presented over time so that family members will have time to become knowledgeable and comfortable with them. They need opportunities to practice the skills in the NICU. Complicated information should be presented clearly and in a variety of ways, with written guidelines for parents to review at a later time. Videos of parents using equipment, monitors and special care techniques should be available for parents via a video lending library.

- Discharge planning should begin early in the infant's hospitalization (Boggs & LaPrade-Wolf, 1992). The plan should be guided by an assessment of family needs regarding care of their infant. The plan should contain elements of the transition plan. Discharge resources should include child care information and parenting guides plus information about how to connect with community, medical follow-up, and family support agencies. Ideally, follow-up instruction and monitoring should be done following discharge.
- "Rooming-in" should be available to parents a few days prior to discharge. This provides parents an opportunity to care for their infant with hospital staff nearby to answer questions and provide support.
- Follow-up clinics should be available for NICU graduates and their families. Clinics should provide follow-up services that include assessment of infant development and health, educational information on infant development and care, assessment of family functioning, and family support via counseling and parent-to-parent groups.

■ SUMMARY

Training and skills considered essential to fostering supportive parent-professional relationships in the NICU include:

- Establishing a communication process that includes listening, empathy and support. As a guide, use such questions as: What is it going to take to relate well with these parents? Do I need to be quiet or assertive? Does this person need emotional support, information, or both?
- Assessing parents' emotional state(s) including, for example, shock, fear, denial and anger. Acknowledge whatever difficulties parents might be having. Understand how emotional states affect communication and parents' level of functioning in the NICU. Parents will range from those who can do much to those who can handle little. Set your expectations accordingly, but seek to involve parents with their infant at whatever level they are able.
- Building on parent competencies. Share your knowledge and skill with the parents in plain talk. Demonstrate positive interventions with infants, for example, comforting and positioning. Encourage parent assistance with the infant.

Do not assume you always need to teach parents; rather, recognize and praise their expertise.

■ Facilitating parents' attachment with their infant. Involve parents with their infant's care plan as soon as possible. Provide information about the infant's signals and behaviors. Emphasize the positive whenever you can.

■ Enabling families to become partners with you, the NICU professional. Work to establish trust, mutual regard and respect with two way communication. Listen to what the parents have to say about their infant. They often know things professionals might have missed or overlooked.

■ Empowering parents through regular reinforcement of their efforts. Let them know that they are more than "only parents." This is a way to help parents gain control and feel involved with their infant's care.

■ Being honest. Do not lie about the facts but be sensitive to the impact your information will have on parents.

■ Making every effort to ensure that parents feel wanted and welcome in the NICU. An infant belongs to its parent(s) and when an infant leaves, it will go home with them. The earlier that parents become involved with you and the infant, the greater chance you have to work together for positive outcomes for the infant.

To plan and implement useful interventions NICU health professionals must examine their own communication, problem solving, and facilitation skills. Because both family and infant states and medical conditions change rapidly, health professionals must recognize changes and help family members understand and deal effectively with change. Comprehensive care includes both medical and psychosocial interventions that empower and enable families in their parenting role.

The time will come when parents and their infant will leave the intensive care unit and enter the larger world. By the time this happens NICU health professionals who practice a family-centered philosophy will have enhanced the understanding and knowledge of parents, taught necessary parenting skills, fostered infant-parent attachment, assisted family coping, helped families understand their own feelings and emotional states, and assisted them in feeling confident and in control. To the extent they have done these things NICU health professionals will have enabled families and NICU graduates to enter their world more securely with a better chance of enhancing the long-term quality of vulnerable babies' lives.

A Place ...

A place of early beginnings
A place of early endings
A place of dreams changed for a lifetime
A place of dreams lost
A place where the struggle for life is so intense
    that you cry within
A place where life's lessons are taught
    by oh, the smallest of teachers
A place where more courage can be witnessed
    in a matter of hours, days, or weeks,
    than can be seen in a lifetime

A place where parent must reach deep within themselves
    just to grasp reality
A place where parents can weep a lifetime of tears
    in a few hours, in a few days
A place where Vanessa, Jeremy, and Dominique
    have passed through and not only have touched
    our hearts but stirred our souls
A place of joy. For after weeks and weeks of obstacles,
    "going home day" is truly a cause for jubilation
A place where the visit of a smiling baby
    gives you the strength to start over again
A place of work...
A place of love.

Anita Gonzales Munguia, RNC
NICU-Neonatal Flight Nurse
(Munguia, 1989)

■ REFERENCES

Able-Boone, H., & Stevens, E. (1994a). After the intensive care nursery experience: Families perceptions of their well-being. *Children's Health Care, 23*, 99–114.

Able-Boone, H., & Stevens, E. (1994b). Family Dynamics and coping after a child's intensive care nursery experience: Implications for early intervention. *Infant-Toddler Intervention, 4*(3), 161–172.

Affleck, G., & Tennen, H. (1991). The effect of newborn intensive care on parents psychological well being. *Children's Health Care, 20*, 6–14.

Affleck, G., Tennen, H., & Rowe, J. (1991). *Infants in crisis: How parents cope with newborn intensive care and its aftermath.* New York: Springer-Verlag.

Arenson, J. (1988). Discharge teaching in the NICU: The changing needs of NICU graduates and their families. *Neonatal Network, 6*, 29–31, 42–52.

Barnard, K. E., C. Snyder, & Spietz, A. (1984). Supportive measures for high-risk infants and their families. In *Social support and families of vulnerable infants* (pp. 291–334). White Plains, NY: March of Dimes Birth Defects Foundation.

Bass, L. S. (1991). What do parents need when their infant is a patient in the NICU? *Neonatal Network, 10,* 25–33.

Benica, S., Longo, C., & Barnsteiner, S. (1992). Perceptions and significances of patient deaths for pediatric critical care nurses. *Critical Care Nurse, 12*(3), 72–75.

Bogdan, R., Brown, M. A., & Foster, S. A. (1982). Be honest but not cruel: Staff-Parent communication on a neonatal unit. *Human Organization, 41,* 6–10.

Boggs, K. U., & LaPrade-Wolf, P. (1992). Beyond survival: Strategies for establishing a follow-up program for infants treated with extracorporeal membrane oxygenation. *Neonatal Network, 11,* 7–13.

Bower, S. A., & Bower, G. H. (1991). *Assert your self.* Reading, MA: Addison-Wesley.

Bruder, M. B., & Cole, M. (1991). Critical elements of transition from NICU to home and follow-up. *Children's Health Care, 20,* 40–49.

Bruder, M. B., & Walker, L. (1990). Discharge planning: Hospital to home transition for infants. *Topics in Early Childhood Special Education, 9,* 26–42.

Cohen, M. R. (1982). Parents' reactions to neonatal intensive care. In R. E. Marshall, C. Kasman, & L. C. Cape (Eds.), *Coping with caring for sick newborns* (pp. 15–30). Philadelphia, PA: W. B. Saunders.

Downey, V. Bengiamin, M., Hever, L., & Juhl, N. (1995). Discharge teaching needs of parents in the NICU. *Neonatal Network, 14*(1), 49–53.

Edwards, K. A., & Allen, M. E. (1988). Nursing management of the human response to premature birth experience. *Neonatal Network, 6,* 82–86.

Ensher, G. L., & Clark, D. A. (1986). Enhancing the potential of parents and infants. Portraits of need and final reflections. In G. L. Ensher & D. A. Clark (Eds.), *Newborns at risk* (pp. 284–304). Rockville, MD: Aspen.

Flynn, L. L., & McCollum, J. (1989). Support systems: Strategies and implication for hospitalized newborns and families. *Journal of Early Intervention, 13,* 173–182.

Frankl, V. (1963). *Man's search for meaning.* New York: Washington Square Press.

Frodi, A., Lamb, M., Leavitt, L., Donovan, M., Neff, L., & Sherry, A. (1978). Fathers' and mothers' responses to the faces and cries of normal and premature infants. *Developmental Psychology, 14,* 490–498.

Gennaro, S. (1985). Maternal anxiety, problem-solving ability and adaptation to the premature infant. *Pediatric Nursing, 11,* 343–348.

Gennaro, S. (1991). Facilitating parenting of the neonatal intensive care graduate. *Journal of Perinatal & Neonatal Nursing, 4,* 55–61.

Gilkerson, L., Gorski, P. A., & Panitz, P. (1990). Hospital-based intervention for preterm infants and their families. In S. J. Meisels & J. P. Sharkoff (Eds.), *Handbook of early childhood interventions* (pp. 445–468). New York: Cambridge University Press.

Goldberg. S., & DiVitto, B. A. (1983). *Born too soon: Premature birth and early delivery.* San Francisco: W.H. Freeman.

Gorski, P. (1987, July). *Parenting needs.* Paper presented at the Developmental Interventions in Neonatal Care Conference. San Francisco, CA.

Greenberg, J. S. (1987). *Comprehensive stress management* (2nd ed.). Dubuque, IA: Wm. C. Brown Publishers.

Griffin, T. (1990). Nurse barriers to parenting in the special care nursery. *Journal of Perinatal and Neonatal Nursing, 4* (2), 56–67.

Grobstein, R. (1982). Innovations in the premature nursery: A survey of parental visiting and related practices. In M. H. Klaus, T. Leger, & M. A. Trause (Eds.), *Maternal attachment and mothering disorders* (pp. 69–71). Skillman, NJ: Johnson & Johnson.

Hanline, M. F., & Deppe, J. (1990). Discharging the premature infant: Family issues and implications for intervention. *Topics in Early Childhood Special Education, 9,* 15–25.

Harrison, H. (1993). The principles for family-centered neonatal care. *Pediatrics, 92,* 643–650.

Harrison, M. J. (1990). A comparison of parental interactions with term and preterm infants. *Research in Nursing & Health, 12,* 173–179.

Haut, C., Peddicord, K., & O'Brien, E. (1994). Supporting parental bonding in the NICU: A care plan for nurses. *Neonatal Network, 13,* 19–25.

Hertzig, M. E., & Mittleman, M. (1984). Temperament in low birthweight children. *Merrill-Palmer Quarterly, 39,* 201–211.

Hughes, M., McCollum, J., Sheffel, D., & Sanchez, G. (1994). How parents cope with the experience of neonatal intensive care. *Children's Health Care, 23,* 1–14.

Jones, C. L. (1982). Environmental analysis of neonatal intensive care. *Journal of Nervous and Mental Disorders, 170,* 130–142.

Krehbiel, R., Munsick-Bruno, G., & Lowe, J. R. (1991). NICU infants born at developmental risk and the individualized family service plan (process) IFSP. *Children's Health Care, 20,* 26–33.

Levy-Schiff, R., Sharir, H., & Mogilner, M. (1987). Mother- and father preterm infant relationship in the hospital preterm nursery. *Child Development, 60,* 93–102.

Londner, R. (1993). Parent-doctor communication: Some ways to close the gap. *NICU News,* March/April, 12–14.

McCluskey-Fawcett, K., O'Brien, M., Robinson, P., & Asay, J. H. (1992). Early transitions for the parents of premature infants: Implications for intervention. *Infant Mental Health Journal, 13,* 147–156.

Mehren, E. (1991). Born too soon. New York: Doubleday.

Miles, M. S., & Carter, M. C. (1985). Coping strategies used by parents during their child's hospitalization in an intensive care unit. *Children's Health Care, 14,* 14–21.

Miles, M. S., Funk, S. G., & Kasper, M. A. (1991). The neonatal intensive care unit environment: Sources of stress for parents. *AACN Clinical Issues in Critical Care Nursing, 2,* 346–354.

Miles, M. S., Funk, S. G., & Kasper, M. A. (1992). The stress response of mothers and fathers of preterm infants. *Research in Nursing & Health, 15,* 261–269.

Miller, S. (1980). Why having control reduces stress. In J. Barber & M. Seligman (Eds.), *Human helplessness: Theory and application* (pp. 71–98). New York: Academic Press.

Munguia, A. G. (1989). A place. *Neonatal Network, 7*, 63.

O'Hare, P. A., & Terry, M. A. (Eds.). (1988). *Discharge planning: Strategies for assuring continuity of care.* Rockville, MD: Aspen.

Oster, A. (1984). Parents of disabled and at risk infants speak to professionals. In *Equals in this partnership* (pp. 26–32). Washington, DC: Maternal and Child Health Clearing House.

Pearl, L., Brown, W., & Myers, M. K. S. (1990). Transition from neonatal intensive care unit: Putting it all together in the community. *Infants and Young Children, 3*, 41–50.

Perehudoff, B. (1990). Parents' perceptions of environmental stressors in the special care nursery. *Neonatal Network, 9*, 39–44.

Plaas, K. M. (1994). The evolution of parental roles in the NICU. *Neonatal Network, 13*, 31-33.

Sabbeth, A. (1984). Marital adjustments to chronic childhood illness: A critique of the literature. *Pediatrics, 73*, 762-767.

Salitross, P. (1986). Transitional infant care: A bridge to home for high risk infants. *Neonatal Network, 4*, 35–41.

Sammons, W. H., & Lewis, J. M. (1985). *Premature babies: A different beginning.* St. Louis: C. V. Mosby.

Schmerber, R. J. (1982). Communication strategies with parents. In *Issues in neonatal care* (pp. 139–146). Chapel Hill, NC: TADS.

Seligman, M. (1975). *Helplessness: On depression, development and death.* San Francisco: Freeman.

Sheikh, L., O'Brien, M., & McCluskey-Fawcett, K. (1993). Parent preparation for the NICU-to-home transition: Staff and parent perceptions. *Children's Health Care, 22*, 227–239.

Stevens, K. R. (1981). Humanistic nursing care for critically ill children. *Nursing Clinics of North America, 16*, 611–622.

Taylor, P. M., & Hall, B. L. (1979). Parents' usual emotional reactions and adjustments to full-term and preterm infants. *Seminars in Perinatology, 3*, 73–89.

Taylor, S. E. (1986). *Health psychology.* New York: Random House.

Thompson, S. (1985. Finding positive meaning in a stressful event and coping. *Basic Applied Social Psychology, 6*, 279–295.

Trause, M. A., & Kramer, L. (1983). The effect of premature birth on parents and their relationships. *Developmental Medicine and Child Neurology, 25*, 459–465.

Vachon, L., & Parkes, E. (1985). Staff stress in the care of the critically ill and dying child. Issues in Comprehensive *Pediatric Nursing, 8*(1–6), 151–182.

Verderber, R. F., & Verderber, K. S. (1995). *Inter-Act: Using interpersonal communication skills* (7th ed.). New York: Wadsworth.

Zeanah, C. H., & Canger, C. I. (1983). The mental health professional in the intensive care nursery. *Zero to Three, 4*, 1–6.

■ CHAPTER 10

Family-Centered Care in the NICU

*The real difficulty in changing the course
of any enterprise lies not in developing
new ideas but in escaping from the old ones.*
John Maynard Keynes

■ INTRODUCTION

The birth and hospitalization of preterm infants bring a bewildering array of emotions and feelings to their families. Parents must make decisions, adjust to new schedules, and face a potentially long and difficult period of separation from their infant. Siblings may see their parents infrequently and be unable to visit their new brother or sister. Grandparents and close family friends may have restricted visiting or none at all. The neonatal intensive unit itself can be stressful to family members who visit their baby in an environment filled with machines and busy professionals caring for very small, sick infants (Haut, Peddicord, & O'Brien, 1994; Thurman & Korteland, 1989).

Families' coping skills are often seriously challenged by their infant's medical crisis (Affleck & Tennen, 1991). The critical care environment may foster less than optimum communication between families and health care professionals at a time when good communication is essential. The NICU experience is often so overwhelming for most families that it remains a vivid, sometimes bittersweet memory long after their infant has been discharged. Here is what one parent had to say:

Families do need nurturing, and I am still angry five-and-a-half years later at the professionals who were too insensitive or unskilled or human to give me what I needed. I am still mad at the doctor who said, when Nick was three days old, that I was in an awfully good mood for someone with a sick baby. I am mad at the nurse who last week told another mother, who called at 11:30 at night to check on her 2 lb.3 oz. son before she went to sleep, that she should call back in an hour, after rounds. The reason that these incidents are worth recalling here is not to prove that, like other people, professionals make mistakes, but because cumulatively their impact on families is profound, and if we care for babies we must meet the needs of families. (Oster, 1984 p. 29)

Because of experiences such as these, a family-centered approach has been developed to frame responses to the birth and hospitalization of preterm infants. The family-centered approach recognizes that the family is a constant in their infant's life. It requires NICU health professionals to respect the parents' role, create opportunities that empower families, and work toward parent/professional collaboration (Wyly & Allen, 1990). The philosophy of family-centered care (FCC) has emerged in response to what parents tell professionals:

- Accept that my child's health care needs are only one part of my family's priorities. Sometimes my family's needs may take precedence.
- Respect my methods of coping without being judgmental.
- Recognize my denial, anger, and fear as natural, healthy grief responses.
- Do not withhold or omit any information concerning the severity or extent of my child's condition.
- Help me understand the range of possibilities.
- Recognize my family's strengths and unique individuality.
- Remind me of my child's strengths from time to time. (Shelton, Jeppson, & Johnson, 1987; Turnbull & Turnbull, 1986).

NICU health professionals recognize the challenge of addressing the needs of families while at the same time attending to the critical needs of infants. While NICUs have been traditionally infant-focused in their care, staff are now looking for ways to support families during hospitalization. They know that neonatal intensive care nurseries do not have to be experienced as alien and stressful. Measures can be taken to minimize the possibility of mixed and conflicting communication. Parents can be helped to experience some control in that environment and consequently feel less stressed. NICU health professionals can work as a team to enable parents to feel more confident with their infant.

Admittedly, providing family-centered care in neonatal intensive care units is difficult. Nonetheless, NICU staff members are exploring family-centered approaches that support families and provide continuity of care (Korteland & Cornwell, 1991; Watterson-Wells, De-Board-Berns, Cook, & Mitchell, 1994). In this chapter we will look at the key elements of family-centered care, at barriers to family-centered care in the NICU, and at ways to overcome these barriers.

FAMILY-CENTERED CARE

Family-centered care stems from the recognition of the pivotal role of the family as the child's primary caregiver. Families are the principal influence on their child's well-being and provide the emotional support and intellectual stimulation needed for the child's optimal development. Further, the family is the primary intermediary between the child and the health care system (McBride, Brotherson, Joanning, Whiddon, & Demmitt, 1993).

The philosophy of family-centered care is based on the family system theory (Minuchin, 1974). Family systems theory recognizes that families are complex, interrelated systems. As systems, families are dynamic and respond adaptively to events that act on them. Experiences that affect an individual family member will affect all of the family. Having an infant in a newborn intensive unit means that the family must make adjustments to the situation. From this perspective, neonatal intensive care should be directed at empowering and enabling families and be responsive to both infant and family priorities (Brown, Thurman, & Pearl, 1993) (see Figure 10–1).

What is family-centered neonatal care? This remains a complex question for both parents and NICU health professionals. Although we do not all agree on how family-centered care should best be implemented, most NICUs recognize the importance of moving in that direction. More attention is being paid to the importance of the family unit and its needs in relation to the medical needs of the premature infant (Rushton, 1990).

The Association for the Care of Children's Health (ACCH) identified nine general principles that recognize the pivotal role of families and thereby underlie the philosophy of family centered care. The major goal of this philosophy is to empower and enable families by supporting their individual needs (Shelton et al., 1987). These principles serve as basic guidelines for family-centered care in the neonatal intensive care unit and are listed in Table 10–1.

While these nine elements of family-centered care outline general standards for providing quality care in the NICU, the methods for adopting and implementing a family-centered approach is still evolving within the context of neonatal intensive care service delivery. In fact, NICU service delivery models are often more infant-centered than family-centered (Brown, Pearl, & Carrasco, 1991). Many questions about neonatal family-centered care are being raised: How

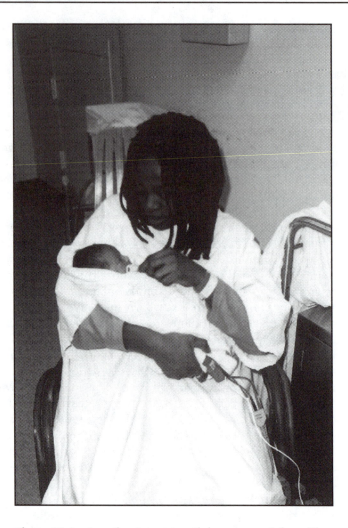

Figure 10–1. A mother interacts with her preterm infant. (Photograph courtesy of Children's Hospital of Buffalo Department of Medical Photography.)

can FCC principles be applied in neonatal intensive care settings? What shifts in orientation must take place to incorporate family members into the critical care setting? What are the limits, if any, to family-centered neonatal care? Despite such questions about implementing FCC in the NICU, many clinicians agree that family-centered care represents "best practice."

TABLE 10–1. Principles of Family-Centered Care

1. Recognizing the family as the constant in the child's life.
2. Facilitating parent/professional collaboration at all stages of health care.
3. Sharing unbiased information with parents about their child's care.
4. Implementing policies that provide emotional and financial support to families.
5. Recognizing family strengths, individuality and different styles of coping.
6. Incorporating the developmental and emotional needs of children into the health delivery system.
7. Encouraging and facilitating parent-to parent support.
8. Assuring that health care delivery is accessible and responsive to family needs.
9. Acknowledging racial, ethnic, cultural and socioeconomic diversity of families.

Family-Centered Neonatal Care

Listen to some family members who have had an infant in the neonatal intensive care nursery:

> "When I first entered the unit, my baby's nurse met me and helped me understand what was being done."

> "After my first visit to the NICU, a representitive from the parent group came to talk with me and asked how the parent group might help."

> "The physician gave us bad news after the first week. I was grateful that she did it in a quiet room away from the nursery."

> "I always felt that I could call to see how my baby was doing."

> "When my son made a turn for the worse, my husband and I had to make a difficult decision about whether to pursue surgery. The physician explained the procedure using terms we could understand. He also described the positive, long term outcomes of surgery. He allowed us time to come to a mutual decision."

These are examples of family-centered neonatal care. Let us look at the principles guiding this approach.

Family-centered neonatal care was the focus of a recent conference of parents and NICU health professionals (Harrison, 1993). The impetus for the conference came from parents of premature infants who believed that NICU staff working collaboratively with families would positively influence infants' care in the NICU. Ten specific principles for family-centered neonatal care were identified. The principles were proposed to help parents and professionals form mutually supportive partnerships in the neonatal intensive care unit and beyond.

1. The basis of family-centered care is open and honest communication between parents and professionals on medical and ethical issues. Policies regarding ethical issues vary from NICU to NICU. Families should be informed of the unit's ethical guidelines as well as the different ethical viewpoints of key NICU health professionals who could determine treatment. Families must make their ethical choices clear to the medical professionals, preferably in writing. They should be decision makers in ethical decisions involving life-support or treatment complications that compromise the infant (Able-Boone, Dokecki, & Smith, 1989).

2. To collaborate with medical professionals in making informed treatment choices, family members must have available the same facts and interpretation of the facts as the medical professionals. The risks and benefits of treatments should be discussed with parents. The communication should not contain medical jargon, but simple, accurate information (Able-Boone et al., 1989). Families need to be accurately informed about their infant's condition and treatment choices. The consequences of experimental or aggressive treatments should be fully elaborated. Experimental treatments and therapies must be fully outlined to parents with information about their safety and efficacy. The medical literature pertaining to their child's condition should be made available to parents.

3. In medical conditions involving considerable risk, aggressive treatment regimens, extensive suffering or very high mortality and morbidity, parents should have the option to make decisions regarding aggressive treatment. Parents and family members need to be informed of the cost-benefit of aggressive treatments. They need to know the differences in medical opinions about proposed treatments and be allowed to choose among accepted treatment options. Parents who do not wish to make such decisions should have the right to designate a physician as their decision maker.

4. Parents who are expecting a baby should be provided information about adverse pregnancy outcomes and given the opportunity to identify treatment options in advance if their infant is born prematurely or critically ill. Under this principle, expectant parents would advise physicians of their preferences for aggressive life support or resuscitation should the need arise. This provides an opportunity for shared decision making between parents and health professionals prior to the infant's birth.

5. Families and medical professionals must work together to recognize and alleviate infant pain in NICUs. Premature infants should not have to endure acute or chronic pain. Pain management should be included in medical protocols in all NICUs. All NICU health professionals should be informed about pain management policies. In the event that pain medication is not recommended for the relief of serious pain, parents must have the option of seeking other medical advice. They must also be decision makers in those medical procedures that may cause their infant acute or chronic pain.

6. Collaborative efforts must be made to reduce unwanted environmental stimuli in the NICU. The brightly lit, often noisy NICU environment creates stress for infants, family members and staff. Working together, parents and staff can make an appropriate environment to facilitate positive infant outcomes and to alleviate family stress.

To improve outcomes, it is recommended that NICU health professionals avoid the routine use of invasive procedures. Unnecessary handling and positioning should be assessed in order to protect babies from sleep disruptions and stress in response to environmental stimuli.

7. Professionals and parents should work together to ensure that new neonatal treatments are safe and have no harmful effects. Controlled evaluations of new treatments are necessary to establish their safety and efficacy. Treatments currently in use that have never been studied should be reexamined using properly controlled trials. Professionals and parents need to advocate neonatal research that is ethical and has scientific validity.

8. Family members should work with NICU health providers to develop policies and programs that encourage maximum involvement of families with their infant. NICUs need to be proactive in systematically promoting parent-to-parent support programs and other parent network groups. Visitation policies should allow open visitation by parents, family members and friends. Any restrictions in the visitation policies should be discussed with parent consultants or parent groups in order to reach a reasonable visitation schedule. Privacy, rooming-in, and breast feeding rooms should be a part of every neonatal unit.

9. Professionals and parents must work collaboratively to promote meaningful long-term follow-up procedures for all high-risk NICU infants. The high percentage of developmental disabilities that occur in very low birthweight (VLBW) infants necessitate both comprehensive long-term follow-up services and available early intervention services. Long-term developmental follow-up is important since many disabilities such as learning and attention disorders do not manifest themselves until after 3 to 4 years of age. Parents need realistic information regarding the development of high-risk infants and the availability of early intervention programs.

10. Both parents and NICU health professionals must recognize that fragile newborns can be harmed by over treatment as well as under treatment. Treatment policies must be based on compassion and the well-being of infants. Adequate support must be made available for NICU survivors with disabilities. Medical treatment of critically ill infants must be done with concern about an infant's long-term outcomes and quality of life. Life-sustaining procedures must be carefully weighed against pain and the infant's welfare. Parents must have more decision-making latitude regarding procedures that promote over treatment and inflict prolonged suffering. Treatment decisions in the NICU must be made with a realistic understanding of available resources for infants with disabilities.

CHANGING PRACTICES IN THE NICU

Beginning in the 1970s NICU caregiving for premature infants began to evolve from an infant-focused to a family-focused model. Today, while most neonatal units embrace family-centered care, in fact, most utilize only components of family-centered care (Brown et al., 1991; O'Brien & Dale, 1994).

Brown et al. (1991) examined the evolution of NICU intervention models. As can be seen in Figure 10–2, the first type of NICU interventions were infant-centered and many studies evaluated the outcomes of tactile and kinesthetic stimulation on the growth and development of premature infants (Kramer, Chamorro, Green, & Knudtson, 1975; Scarr-Salapatek & Williams, 1973; White & Labarba, 1976).

In the 1980s, NICU interventions began to emphasize individualized infant assessment, appropriate developmental care for the sick premature infant, and facilitation of parent-infant interactions. Studies of NICU-based parent self-help groups (Minde et al., 1980) and of systematic training on infant abilities and development (Widmayer & Field, 1981) found that both interventions enhanced the quantity and quality of parent-infant interactions.

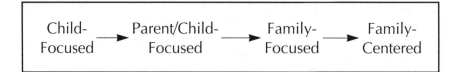

Child-Focused → Parent/Child-Focused → Family-Focused → Family-Centered

Figure 10–2. Evolution of NICU intervention models. (From Brown, W., Pearl, L. F., & Carrasco, N. [1991]. Evolving models of family-centered services in neonatal intensive care. *Children's Health Care, 20*, 50–55. Reprinted with permission.)

Brown et al. (1980) examined the short- and long-term effects of mothers' involvement with their infants in the NICU. Although a number of outcome measures were used, the only difference between intervention and comparison group mothers was that intervention group mothers visited their babies more often while the mothers themselves were still hospitalized. From this early research came NICU intervention models that emphasized positive parent-infant interactions to improve infant development. Visitation policies were changed to facilitate more family involvement (Plaas, 1994). O'Brien and Dale (1994) point out that the research studies which focused on parental involvement in infant care typically focused on infants rather than on the family system.

Elements of family-centered neonatal care began to be more systematically examined in the 1980s and 1990s. Researchers investigated how providing personal support to parents reduced parental stress. A formal support program designed to assist mothers' transition from the NICU to home care of their infants (Affleck, Tennen, Rowe, Roscher, & Walker, 1989). Some mothers indicated that they did not want or need a support program. For those mothers who indicated they needed the most support, their participation in the support program positively affected their sense of competence, perceived control, and responsiveness.

Two different coping interventions were studied regarding how well they helped mothers of preterm infants manage the stress of their infants' hospitalization. Training in active problem-focused coping strategies and in emotion-focused strategies designed to manage anxiety were found to reduce anxiety and lessen depression in mothers of NICU infants (Corbiella, Mabe, & Forehand, 1990).

Parker, Zahr, Cole, and Brecht (1992) tested a NICU intervention program that included training, education, and support for low-SES mothers in the NICU. The intervention was designed to enhance their skills at providing a stimulating and emotionally supportive environment for their premature infants. The intervention group, compared to the control group, had higher scores on the Bayley Scales of Infant Development at 4 and 8 months corrected age (Bayley, 1969). The HOME scale was used to measure the quality of the home environment (Caldwell & Bradley, 1979).

Several family-centered neonatal programs were funded as 3-year model-demonstration projects by the Handicapped Children's Early Education Program (HCEEP), Office of Special Education Programs. Evaluations of the programs' effectiveness are currently being completed. Two of those projects are described below.

The LIFT (Liaison Infant Family Team Project) project was based on an ecological systems approach aimed at promoting supportive relationships between infants and their families in the NICU (Thurman, Cornwell, & Korteland, 1989). The program, jointly administered by Bryn Mawr Hospital and Temple University from 1986–1989, was designed to provide family-centered services in a neonatal intensive care unit by providing support services that empowered families and promoted an adaptive fit within the family. Services were provide based on individual family needs. A case study analysis of the effectiveness of the LIFT project is now underway. Results to date indicate that if NICUs want to provide family-centered care, they must be adaptive and serve as facilitators of plans and services (VandenBerg & Hanson, 1993).

The Ecological Caregiving for Home Outcomes (ECHO) project was a 3-year HCEEP model demonstration project located in Johnson City, Tennessee. The program goals were to develop, implement, and evaluate a family-centered care model that began in the NICU and transitioned to the community. The five program components were: (1) newborn child-find procedures, (2) linkage to early intervention services, (3) five-level range of service, (4) developmental intervention and family support in the NICU, and (5) transition facilitation. Evaluation of the program's components is currently underway.

There is a paucity of research on efforts to implement and evaluate family-centered neonatal services. Components of family-centered care such as family support and parent-to-parent networks are being incorporated in NICUs, yet systematic controlled studies have yet to be done. Given the extensive literature on the impact of prematurity on the family system, there is a clear need to carry out well-designed, data-based studies that evaluate family-centered interventions in the NICU.

BARRIERS TO FAMILY-CENTERED CARE

The family-centered approach is based on a new philosophy of care which has been identified as a shift in paradigm (Kuhn, 1970; Thurman, 1991). Turnbull and Summers (1985) likened it to a "Copernican Revolution" when Copernicus stated that the earth revolved around the sun rather than the sun revolving around the earth. The revolution of family-centered care puts the family and infant in the center of the universe with the health care delivery service revolving around it.

Actual NICU practices and policies are not always congruent with a family-centered philosophy. Often health care providers are frustrated with the idea of what family-centered care is and with how it is implemented in a critical care setting. Some doubt that it is possible to provide family support and empowerment in an intensive care unit.

What needs to be done to implement family-centered care in the NICU? Let us first examine some of the barriers to family-centered care in the NICU. First, there are barriers that need to be overcome. They may vary from unit to unit depending on a hospital's organizational structure and philosophical commitment to families.

Medical Training Priorities

There is widespread recognition that families with infants in the NICU experience stress as a result of their infant's hospitalization (McCluskey-Fawcett, O'Brien, Robinson, & Asay, 1992). The overwhelming events associated with having a high-risk infant in the NICU affects all family members. Providing emotional support, responding to the needs of families, and helping them in the decision-making process are interventions that can have a positive impact on the entire family system (Arrango, 1990).

Integrating families into the care of their infant involves acceptance of the principles of family-centered care (Thurman, 1991). For medical staff who have been trained to focus on infant care, incorporating family-centered care into NICU practices represents a major philosophical shift. For example, the needs of families in the context of critical care may not be perceived as valuable or even useful, and NICU staff may not accept the idea that interventions that encompass both infants and families are as effective as infant-focused interventions.

Rushton (1990) points out that the training priorities of NICU staff may not reflect family-centered priorities. Training may focus on technology, new medical procedures, and medications rather than on interaction and communication skills with families.

Critical Care Approach

One barrier to family-centered care is that the critical function of neonatal intensive care units is to save infants' lives. A substantial portion of preterm infants' hospitalization is acute care. Infants in this phase are often critically ill and require ventilator support. They go from one medical crisis to another. During this critical care phase, the support that families need is not always available because staff must focus on the needs of the critically ill infant. In some NICUs, family-centered care begins around the time the infant becomes stabilized. In other units, family needs are attended to only during preparation for discharge which can be weeks or months after the infant's admission. When this is the case, family members have had to cope, largely by themselves, with a critical and frightening situation that may extend over a period of months (Gilkerson, Gorski, & Panitz, 1990).

Staff Attitudes

The attitudes of staff who are committed to infant-focused care can be impediments to family-centered care. Attitudes often associated with traditional medically focused training may result in staff who are unwilling to involve family members in developmental interventions or nonmedical care. NICU health care professionals may doubt parents' ability to contribute to routine caregiving such as diapering or bathing. Involving family members in such activities may be perceived as adding to an already overwhelming work load. Other NICU professionals may feel that the while the infant is hospitalized, they are the exclusive caregivers. You see signs of this when professionals use terms such as "my baby" which can create competition between parents and professionals.

Families' visits may be viewed as distracting or unwanted. Further, staff attitudes regarding visitation may be translated into restricted visiting policies. NICUs, for example, may convey an unwelcome atmosphere toward families by posting signs that inform family members what hours they cannot visit and by not supplying comfortable chairs next to infants' isolettes.

Collaborating with family members on important decisions concerning their infant's care may be viewed as unnecessary, since the staff view themselves as the experts. Some professionals fear a loss of control if they involve family members in decision making. Others may doubt parents' ability to make reasonable decisions while stressed by having a critically ill infant.

Staff attitudes about their work may also distance them from families. NICU professionals may feel that under all circumstances they must be the expert on every aspect of an infant's care, even when they doubt their own knowledge or skill in a specific area. Some neonatal nurses label this the "imposter syndrome" (Wyly, 1993). It is, of course, unrealistic to assume that NICU health professionals can be experts at all times in the rapidly changing NICU world. These attitudes, however, create stress for the NICU professionals as well as barriers when parents pose difficult questions or ask about new procedures.

Family-centered care can also be inhibited when staff members assume responsibility for patient outcomes that are out of their control. High expectations for successful outcomes and feelings of failure when they do not occur can create tension between parents and professionals (Rushton, 1990).

Collectively, these attitudes serve to isolate families in a situation that they already find to be alien. Family involvement with their infant may decrease rather than increase. The overall experience for families, even after their infants are discharged, can be negative.

Equipment and Technology

The equipment and technology required in an acute care setting can also be a impediment to family-centered care. NICU professionals must constantly keep pace with the demands of the rapidly changing technology. The time required to learn how to use new equipment often means that less time can be devoted to family needs. The high-technology nature of the NICU also places barriers to communication with families by distancing them from NICU caregivers. Family members who follow the model of the health professional may in turn focus on the equipment and application of treatments and thus pay less attention to the developmental needs of their infant.

Communication

How NICU staff communicate with families and each other can be an impediment to family-centered neonatal care. Effective communication is lost when staff do not appear to be willing to listen and hear what family members are saying. Professionals are often unaware that their use of medical jargon, acronyms, and abbreviations can confuse parents attempting to adjust to the intensive care setting. If procedures and infant progress are explained using complex medical terminology, an opportunity to engage the family is lost.

Parents report that communication problems arise when their infant's primary caregiver identifies the baby by the wrong name or sex. Mehren (1991), a parent of a premature girl, described this exchange with her baby's neonatologist:

> "I'll be drawing blood from him and having it sent down to the lab," Dr. Ho told me.
>
> "Her," I said.
>
> Through his thick, wire-rimmed glasses, Dr. Ho gave me a blank look.
>
> "Her," I said. "You'll be drawing more blood from her. Emily is a girl, not a boy. Have you noticed?"
>
> Now Dr. Ho tossed me an expression of disgust. "We call all the babies 'he,'" he said. "It's less complicated." (Mehren, 1991, p. 117)

Because NICUs are often crowded, busy places, parents who visit their infants often overhear staff talking to one another. Angry, confrontive communication between staff members can intimidate parents and make the NICU even more threatening than it might be. Staff who use derogatory terms for babies in the nursery, may be heard by family members. Terms such as "rug-rat," "toaster-head," or "bad boy/girl" convey the message that infants are not perceived as individuals or even human by staff. When staff use expressions such as "bag the baby," "baby had a spell," "Braydies," or "trainwreck" they run the risk of being misunderstood and may even frighten parents.

Staffing

When NICUs are understaffed, as is so often the case, staff members feel overwhelmed by the increased demands of their workload. Neonatal nurses often describe a 12-hour shift where there is no time for breaks or meals because of the ongoing crises that require their continuous attention (Wyly, 1993). This results in increased staff stress and exhaustion. In such situations staff may have little time to provide comfort and support to parents or to involve them in their child's care.

Few NICUs have a full-time, family-centered professional or a paid parent advocate because funds have not been allocated for such roles. This reflects the organization's priorities regarding family-focused care. When such positions do exist, how they function within the intensive care setting is often unclear. For example, will family-centered professionals be called into the unit by nurses or physicians, will they be available in the unit on an ongoing basis, or will their function differ from the function of social workers assigned to the unit?

Other Barriers

There are other potential impediments to family-centered neonatal services. NICUs in which there are no clear lines of authority for developing and implementing family-focused care may hinder family-centered NICU care. The NICU's physical layout may preclude family privacy. Small, overcrowded neonatal intensive care units may not have space for parents to sit and comfortable family waiting rooms may be missing. The unit's organization may focus on acute care rather than on chronic care despite the current reality that NICUs must meet the needs of both acutely and chronically ill infants.

Staff training that omits skills needed to provide family supportive interventions pose still another barrier to practices in family-centered services. Many families of high-risk infants need to be linked to services beyond the NICU. NICUs that do not provide continuity of care throughout hospitalization, discharge, and after discharge lack an essential element in family focused care.

IMPLEMENTING FAMILY-CENTERED NEONATAL CARE

Working with families in the NICU presents many challenges for health professionals who are oriented toward the critical care that maximizes an infant's chance of survival. Although an infant focus is necessary, support for families is often not available. Family-centered neonatal care is an innovative approach to ensure family support in the NICU with transition continuity to the community. The FCC model fosters partnership and collaborative growth among families and NICU health providers without de-emphasizing the medical and developmental needs of the infant (Institute for Family-Centered Care, 1994). Thus the family-centered approach, which includes care for both infant and family, is broader than the traditional infant-centered focus (McBride et al., 1992).

Family centered-care supports families in their role as caregiver (Thurman, 1993). Among all the activities in the NICU, the experience that parents remember most is the amount and kind of support they received from health providers (Sosnowitz, 1984). The FCC philosophy views families as partners in the health care of their child. This partnership requires health professionals to communicate with families, to recognize individual family strengths, and to involve them in decision making and various aspects of their child's care (Holloway, 1994).

How can family-centered neonatal services be implemented in the NICU? What changes in resources and training will facilitate this care model? Thurman (1991) suggests four principles to guide family centered-care services in the NICU:

1. Establish and maintain adaptive fit within the family and between the family system and the service delivery system.
2. Provide services based on family identified needs and desires.
3. Foster family independence and empowerment while providing a stable ongoing support system.
4. Recognize that families are complex, dynamic and ever changing systems.

These principles require NICUs to reexamine their philosophy of care, organization and service delivery expectations. Let us examine some strategies for implementing family-centered care in the neonatal intensive care unit.

NICU Self-Study

The first step in incorporating a family-centered NICU model is to conduct a rigorous self-study of the NICU organization, philosophy, staff attitudes, and policies. The self-study should include self-reports, questionnaires, and a review of current procedures and policies. Focus groups composed of staff, administrators and parents of NICU graduates should address the following questions.

- Are our policies flexible and responsive to both infant and family needs?
- What are the procedures for changing NICU policies? Are they adaptable?
- In what ways is our NICU environment conducive/not conducive to building trusting relationships and ensuring collaboration with families?
- How does the authority structure of the unit match the decision making structure?
- Who makes the decisions?
- What is our current conceptual framework and philosophy regarding families of infants?
- How do we involve families in decision making?
- What are the ways we collaborate with family members on nonmedical developmental care of their infant?
- How do we communicate information to families?
- How are ethical decisions made in the NICU?
- What is the climate of our unit in terms of our tolerance of plurality of beliefs and viewpoints?
- What are the prevailing staff attitudes regarding family support, involvement, and family-centered care?
- How does our NICU environment promote/not promote an atmosphere that is welcoming and invites family collaboration?
- What is our high turnover rate and how does it relate to worker stress?
- What is our visitation policy?

A self-study allows the institution to carefully examine the policies and climate that characterizes the NICU. Policies, staff priorities and attitudes that may impede family-centered care can be identified. Ways to overcome obstacles to family-centered care can be discussed. A self-study allows an in-depth look at the family-centered procedures currently in place. A well-designed self-study should provide direction about how to develop policies and procedures that both match individual NICUs and facilitate staff responsiveness to family needs.

Currently, the Institute for Family-Centered Care is preparing a self assessment inventory (Newborn Intensive Care Units: A Self-Assessment Inventory) for NICU staff to assess family-centered care practices and policies in their units (Johnson, 1995, personal communication). This assessment is designed to be used with an interdisciplinary NICU team including families. The checklist is to be used as a tool to promote discussion among team members about family-centered neonatal care.

The success of implementing FCC depends in large part on the willingness of the hospital and NICU to commit to families (Vestal & Richardson, 1981). The administration must document the change process and identify the components that are lacking and that promote FCC. Teams of administrators, staff, and parents working toward the goal of family-centered services can provide leadership by establishing a FCC network within the hospital to promote change. Overall, staff members should be guided by the question "To become family-centered, what changes must I make in my practice?"

Staff Training

Staff training and development is essential when implementing family-centered care. Training should encompass several components (Table 10–2). One training component should focus on the essentials of family-centered care. Included should be (1) effective communication skills, (2) the impact of premature birth on the family system and family emotional states, (3) strategies for providing emotional support in the NICU, and (4) ways to collaborate with family members on developmental care and decision making.

TABLE 10-2. Family-Centered Neonatal Care Staff Training Components

- Effective communication skills
- Impact of premature birth on families
- Emotional support strategies
- Involving families in developmental care
- Ways to promote family collaboration and decision making
- Team building
- Providing continuity of care from NICU to home
- Applying developmentally appropriate infant interventions
- Modify the NICU environment to support infant/parents
- Resources on Public Law 99-457

One example of a family-centered training model is the NICU Training Project which trains NICU health providers in team building, collaboration for family-centered care, ways to incorporate family members in developmental care, and the use of effective communications with family members. Role plays, simulations, and case study analysis are used in the training to sensitize NICU staff to the family's NICU experience. For example, staff trainees write a developmental care plan for specific infants in their care and then discuss ways to use the plan as a communication tool with parents and to involve parents in updating it (Wyly, Allen, Pfalzer, & Wilson, 1993).

Continuity of care from admission to the NICU through discharge to home is another important training component. Coordinated service systems that facilitate families' link to community services should begin in the neonatal intensive care unit. Training should address ways to assist families in transition from the NICU, for example, discharge plans and parent education.

NICU staff need resources regarding information about Public Law 99-457 that ensures care for infants with special needs or disabilities. Under this law, such infants and their families are eligible for family-centered developmental services beginning during hospitalization (Krehbiel, Munsick-Bruno, & Lowe, 1991). Public Law 99-457 requires a written document called the Individual Family Service Plan (IFSP) that indicates goals and suggested services. The IFSP process and ongoing family-centered activities including discharge and transition from hospital to home should be included as part of staff training.

A third training focus encompasses team building and ways that interdisciplinary teams can work together to support family members in the NICU. Strategies that help interdisciplinary team members work together should be identified. For example, a physical therapist might work with a parent and a nurse to assess the optimum positioning of a very fragile infant. Collaborative efforts should be demonstrated to alleviate work overload in the NICU.

A fourth training focus involves assisting neonatal health professionals to recognize infants' developmental milestones and how such milestones are altered in high-risk hospitalized infants. Attention must be paid to developmentally appropriate interventions with acute and chronic infants. Ways to assess infant cues and behaviors, initiating individualized developmental care, and involving family members in developmental care are necessary parts of the training.

A fifth focus involves strategies for change in the NICU. Changing the NICU environment to support families and infants should be outlined including ways that staff can provide a more welcoming environment. Policy and administrative changes that can be implemented for family-centered care can be planned by staff.

The training process must be carefully designed to change existing attitudes and to facilitate the acquisition of skills and knowledge. Administrators must support staff training at all levels. The training plan should employ current state-of-the art training techniques that enhance adult learning. To maximize training effectiveness the training should promote active learning through case studies, demonstrations, simulations, role plays, and learning designs that refine problem-solving skills. Training follow-up on the use of the methods and information is a part of effective training. Moreover, training outcomes should be assessed by measuring and documenting attitude and behavioral changes.

Parent-to-Parent Support

A key element in family-centered care is parent-to-parent support. NICUs can facilitate parent support groups as well as link families to veteran parents of NICU graduates. Some NICUs provide a social worker, psychologist, or parent advocate to work with parents to organize parent support groups. Parent Care Inc., (9041 Colgate Street, Indianapolis, IN 46428-1210) a national organization of parents and professionals, links NICU parent support groups throughout the United States and provides guidelines for organizing parent support organizations.

Parent groups can help families feel less isolated and provide empathy and understanding (Winch & Christoph, 1988). Parent support groups help parents cope more effectively during crises (Hughes, McCollum, Sheftel, & Sanchez, 1994; Nathanson, 1986). Their shared similar experiences in the NICU foster problem solving and new approaches concerned with issues of infant hospitalization.

In addition to sharing feelings through group work, some parent groups provide services such as taking pictures of the infants as a gift to new parents. Others make bereavement clothes for infants who die. Still others offer assistance and information on the family's first NICU visit. There is no question that parent-to-parent support is a rich, often under-used means of meeting the psychosocial needs of families in the NICU. Neonatal intensive care units that encourage parent support groups are strengthening their family-centered care services.

EARLY INTERVENTION IN THE NICU

Congress passed an amendment to the 1975 Education for All Handicapped Children Act (PL 99-142). This amendment, known as Public Law 99-457 Part H, extended the age range of free public education from birth to 5 years for infants and children with disabilities. The law specifically says that states are "to develop and implement a statewide, comprehensive, coordinated, multidisciplinary, interagency program of early intervention services for handicapped infants and toddlers and their families" (Section 61b). This means that the hospital is now included as an early intervention site.

The family-centered philosophy identified by the Association for the Care of Children's Health (Johnson, McGonigel, & Kaufmann, 1989) is congruent with the intent of Public Law 99-457. The principles of family-centered care include family-professional collaboration, support of family needs, respect for differences in ethnic and cultural diversity, and promotion of family decision making.

Under PL 99-457 many infants in the NICU are considered eligible for early intervention services. Depending on a state's criteria for developmental disabilities, those infants eligible for early intervention are those with known disabilities such as Down syndrome or cerebral palsy, as well as infants at-risk for developmental problems, for example, intraventricular hemorrhage, very low birthweight, adolescent parents, and respiratory distress syndrome.

Infants and their families who qualify may elect to receive early intervention services delivered by an interdisciplinary team that includes special educators, physical therapists, psychologists, occupational therapists, speech and language therapists, and the infant's parents. Other professionals such as neonatal nurses, physicians, social workers, and respiratory therapists may be included when early intervention services begin in the NICU.

Traditionally, early intervention component of services began sometime after the infant's discharge. Currently, efforts are being made to provide early intervention assistance for infants born at-risk for development and with identified developmental concerns in the NICU (Krehbiel et al., 1991; Wyly, Allen, Pfalzer, & Wilson, 1993).

Individualized Family Service Plan

Under PL 99-457 early intervention services are available and designed to meet the individual needs of the infant and family. Early intervention services include any activity that promotes the infant/family outcomes identified in the Individualized Family Service Plan (IFSP) (Table 10–3). The IFSP guides the early intervention services and is product of collaboration between professionals and families. The IFSP is designed to empower and enable families by identifying their needs and strengths.

The IFSP is a legal written document. It is not necessarily long but must contain the information specified in Table 10–3. The process of developing and implementing the IFSP is considered to be more

TABLE 10–3.   Content of the IFSP

∎ Description of the child's present level of development including cognitive, language and speech, psychosocial, physical development, and self-help skills; a statement of strengths and needs. The developmental profile must be based on acceptable objective criteria.

∎ If the family agrees, a statement of the family strengths and needs related to optimizing their infants development.

∎ A statement of major outcomes expected to be achieved for the child and family, including the criteria, procedures, and timelines and whether revisions of the outcomes are necessary.

∎ A statement of specific early intervention services necessary to meet the unique needs of child and family, including frequency, intensity, and method of delivering services.

∎ The projected dates for initiation of services and the anticipated duration of services.

∎ The name of the case manager from the profession most immediately relevant to the child's or family's needs who will be responsible for implementing and coordinating services.

∎ The steps to be taken to support the transition of the child to services provided under part B of the Act if appropriate.

valuable than the IFSP product. The approach to developing an IFSP respects family autonomy and independence while developing best practice for early intervention services (NEC*TAS and ACCH, 1989). The IFSP document represents a product of family-centered care in the NICU wherein NICU professionals, family members, and early interventionists work together to build on family and infant strengths while recognizing the unique needs of individual families. How can the IFSP process be integrated into the NICU? This is a new endeavor which requires NICUs to examine their attitudes and philosophy about family centered care. Let us look at some ways the components of the IFSP process might be integrated into the neonatal intensive care setting.

Infant's Present Level of Development

NICU health professionals can use naturalistic observations of fragile preterm infants in the unit to assess development, for example, the Assessment of Preterm Infant Behavior (APIB) scale designed to evaluate the developmental function of high-risk infants (Als, 1982). As premature infants grow and become more stable the Brazelton

Neonatal Assessment Scale (BNAS) can be used to assess behavioral and neurologic function in infants (Brazelton, 1973).

Statement of Family Strengths and Needs

The family needs and strengths can be reported by family members via a family "diary" kept by family members during their infant's hospitalization. The diary would contain their changing priorities of infant care during the NICU stay, identify their unique coping styles, their support systems, and their hopes for their baby.

Krehbiel et al. (1991) suggest that NICU staff use open-ended family interviews to identify family supports, fears, visiting routines, ways of coping, and specific needs. Information gathering should take place over time with respect for families' emotional states and grieving. The process of gathering this information should be supportive and enhance family member's self-confidence for caring for a high-risk infant.

Outcomes Expected for Infant and Family

When the IFSP is first written the interdisciplinary team identifies three or four infant/family outcomes. These are updated or changed as the need arises. An outcome can focus on any infant developmental area or aspect of family functioning that the family thinks will optimize their infant's development. The IFSP outcomes are written in terms of what is to occur and what is expected when it occurs. For example:

Infant Outcome: To allow Lisa practice in using normal self-comforting behaviors, her hand will be positioned close to her mouth. It is expected that sucking on her hand will occur in responses to changes in her environmental stimulation.

Family Outcome: Mr. and Mrs. Brown want to learn more about John's feeding problems and ways to manage them as they assume responsibility for his feeding. They will be contacted by the feeding specialist who will demonstrate oral stimulation techniques that facilitate infant feeding. It is expected that the parents will be able to feed John successfully at home.

These outcome statements are written collaboratively by parents and professionals. While professionals share their expertise, family members share their knowledge and experience to reach an agreed upon goal. The process reflects shared planning and decision making.

In conclusion, IFSPs can be written while the infant is hospitalized in the NICU. It supports families with infants with disabilities in the NICU and through transition to community-based early intervention services.

Providing Early Intervention Services

Early intervention services in the NICU include any activity that addresses the needs of infant and family. These services are individualized based on the assessment of infant and family. As family and infant needs change the IFSP needs to be modified. According to PL 99-457 these changes are done by an interdisciplinary team that includes the parents. In the NICU, daily or weekly rounds or family-staff meetings can be vehicles for this process.

Examples of specific intervention services for infants might include positioning and handling, feeding protocols, or provision of certain types of sensory stimulation. To provide consistency of care across caregivers, Cole, Begish-Duddy, Judas, and Jorgensen (1990) recommend the use of a developmental care plan which identifies the strengths, stressors, and developmental needs of infants. The care plan can be updated by parents and staff and posted at the infant's bedside. It can also be used as a transition tool when the infant is discharged from the NICU to home. See Figure 10–3 for an example of a developmental care plan.

Family interventions may include linking family members to parent support groups, parenting classes, case management, or grief counseling. Services that address stated family needs should be identified such as respite services, child care, and transportation to and from the hospital.

The projected start dates of early intervention services vary as a function of the medical status of the infant and the family's readiness to begin intervention. For very fragile infants the IFSP process might be delayed until the infant is stable and parents are able to participate. In the case of infants who are relatively healthy, the process might begin a few days after admission.

Case management is mandated by PL 99-457. The case manager is accountable for implementing the IFSP process and coordinating the interdisciplinary team. The case manager ensures that the IFSP process promotes family capacities and competencies to obtain needed resources and services. The case manager is named from the profession most immediately relevant to the infant or family's needs. The case manager must be trained in case management and should be family-centered in approach. An important function of the case manager is that of linking families to resources and facilitating transition. NICUs are now identifying personnel to serve as case managers in the NICU.

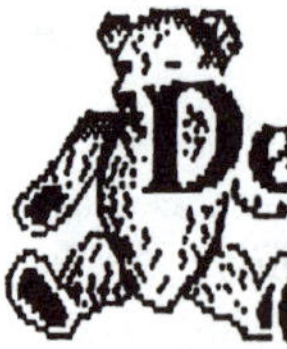

Figure 10–3. Sample Developmental Care Plan. (Adapted from Cole, J. G., Begish-Duddy, A., Judas, M. L., & Jorgensen, K. M. (1990). Changing the NICU environment: The Boston City Hospital Model. *Neonatal Network, 9*, 15–22.)

Another component of early intervention is transition out of the NICU to home or another facility. Most families with infants who have been identified at developmental risk will require early intervention services from community agencies. This requires comprehensive coordination of care from hospital to home which includes linking families to primary service providers in the community. Transition planning should be ongoing during the infant's hospitalization. Parents and other family members should have access to information and support to enable them to feel confident in the care of their infant at home. The discharge process must promote continuity of care and respond to the needs of the parents (Drake, 1995).

As service providers and parents look for ways to improve the life circumstances of the high-risk infant in the NICU, there must be efforts made to train personnel to cooperatively meet the challenges of this new field (VandenBerg, 1987). Public Law 99-457 mandates a comprehensive, coordinated, multidisciplinary, interagency approach for serving very young infants. This service requires cooperation between hospitals and early intervention service programs.

Clinicians and investigators recognize the need to train NICU and early intervention professionals to work with premature infants with disabilities and their families to provide appropriate development of intervention and family support. Cooper and Kennedy (1989) wrote:

> Advances in neonatal intensive care have dramatically increased the survival rate of infants born prematurely or with medical complications. Figures show that the number of neonatal intensive care units (NICUs) in the United States increased from 448 to 594 in 1985 (Hospital Statistics, 1987). Increases in infant survival rates, coupled with the enactment of 99-457, have created a necessity for professionals involved with infant service delivery to have up-to-date knowledge concerning neonatal intensive care.... Consequently, the infant interventionist must be well acquainted with the treatment approaches utilized in the NICU. (Cooper & Kennedy, 1989, p. 33)

To address these needs, Miller, Mutton, and Williams (1993) tested a collaborative training program in which early childhood special education students rotated through a level three NICU for 15–20 hours. Student learners gained an understanding of the experiences of preterm infants and their families. The NICU staff gained a greater understanding of community-based early intervention programs.

An interdisciplinary training program was implemented and evaluated by Wyly et al. (1993). NICU-based health providers and early intervention professionals are brought together for two days of training. The training focus is on continuity of intervention from NICU to home, family-centered care, and team collaboration. As a result of training, participating neonatal units have identified procedures for family-focused care and linkage with early intervention agencies.

SUMMARY

Although NICUs endorse the concept of family-centered care, only a few actually implement FCC practices. One reason for this is the lack of consensus among NICU professionals and parents on what family-centered neonatal care is.

The philosophy of family-centered care recognizes the pivotal role of the family in the child's care and development. Further, family-centered care entails a partnership between professionals and families and recognition that every family is unique and has strengths. In the NICU, family-centered care expands the critical care for infants to include family-oriented interventions NICU health professionals must recognize the barriers to FCC and find ways to overcome them. Some barriers to family-centered neonatal services are staff resistance to family involvement, staff attitudes that reflect work as exclusively infant-focused, technology, organizational philosophy, communication issues, and under-staffing.

Successful implementation of family-centered services in the NICU requires many changes. Hospitals and NICUs must systematically examine their attitudes and commitment to families so that administration, staff, and families can identify areas of needed change and then work together to implement the changes. Staff training and development are needed to provide information and to achieve attitude and behavior changes. NICUs must facilitate parent-to-parent support and recognize its contribution to the successful implementation of family-centered care.

REFERENCES

Able-Boone, H., Dokecki, P. R., & Smith, M. S. (1989). Parent and health care provider communication and decision making in the intensive care nursery. *Children's Health Care, 18*(3), 133–141.

Affleck, G., Tennen, H., Rowe, J., Roscher, B., & Walker, L. (1989). Effects of formal support on mothers' adaption to the hospital-to-home transition of high-risk infants: The benefits and costs of helping. *Child Development, 60*, 488–501.

Affleck, G., & Tennen, H. (1991). The effect of newborn intensive care on parents' psychological well-being. *Children's Health Care, 20*, 6–14.

Als, H. (1982). Toward a synactive theory of development: Promise for the assessment and support of infant individuality. *Infant Mental Health Journal, 3*, 229–243.

Arrango, P. (1990). A parent's perspective: "Family-centered care": Making it a reality. *Children's Health Care, 19*, 57–62.

Bayley, N. (1969). *The Bayley Scales of Infant Development*. New York: Psychological Corporation.

Brazelton, T. B. (1973). Neonatal behavioral assessment scale. *Clinics in Developmental Medicine #88*. Philadelphia, PA: J. B. Lippincot.

Brown, J. V., LaRussa, M. M., Aylward, G. P., Davis, D. J., Rutherford, P. K., & Bakeman, R. (1980). Nursery-based intervention with prematurely born babies and their mothers: Are there effects? *Journal of Pediatrics, 97*, 487–491

Brown, W., Pearl, L. F., & Carrasco, N. (1991). Evolving models of family-centered services in neonatal intensive care. *Children's Health Care, 20,* 50–55.

Brown, W., Thurman, S. K., & Pearl, L. F. (1993). *Family-centered early interventions with infants & toddlers: Innovative cross-disciplinary approaches.* Baltimore: Paul H. Brookes Publishing.

Caldwell, B., & Bradley, R (1979). *Home Observation for Measurement of the Environment.* Little Rock, AR: University of Arkansas.

Cole, J. G., Begish-Duddy, A., Judas, M. L., & Jorgensen, K. M. (1990). Changing the NICU environment: The Boston City Hospital Model. *Neonatal Network, 9*(2), 15–22.

Cooper, C. S., & Kennedy, R. D. (1989). An update for professionals working with neonates at risk. *Topics in Early Childhood Special Education, 9,* 32–50.

Corbiella, C. W., Mabe, P. A., & Forehand, R. L. (1990). A comparison of two stress-reduction treatments for mothers of neonates hospitalized in a neonatal intensive care unit. *Children's Health Care, 19,* 93–100.

Drake, E. (1995). Discharge teaching needs of parents in the NICU. *Neonatal Network, 14,* 49–53.

Gilkerson, L., Gorski, P. A., & Panitz, P. (1990). Hospital-based intervention for preterm infants and their families. In S. J. Meisels & J. P. Sharkoff (Eds.), *Handbook of early childhood interventions* (pp. 445–448). New York: Cambridge University Press.

Haut, C., Peddicord, K., & O'Brien, E. (1994). Supporting parental bonding in the NICU: A plan for nurses. *Neonatal Network, 8,* 19–25.

Harrison, H. (1993). The principles for family-centered neonatal care. *Pediatrics, 92,* 643–650.

Holloway, E. (1994). Parent and occupational therapist collaboration in the neonatal intensive care unit. *The American Journal of Occupational Therapy, 48,* 535–538.

Hughes, M., McCollum, J., Sheftel, D., & Sanchez, G. (1994). How parents cope with the experience of neonatal intensive care. *Children's Health Care, 23,* 1–14.

Institute for Family Centered Care (1994). Essential allies: Families and professionals working together to improve quality of care. *Advances in Family Centered Care, 1,* 1.

Johnson, B., McGonigel, M., & Kaufman, R. (1989). *Guidelines and recommended practices for the individualized family service plan.* Washington, DC: National Early Childhood Technical Assistance System and Association for the Care of Children's Health.

Korteland, C., & Cornwell, J. T. (1991). Evaluating family-centered programs in neonatal intensive care. *Children's Health Care, 20,* 56–61.

Kramer, M., Chamorro, I., Green, D., & Knudtson, F. (1975). Extra tactile stimulation of the premature infant. *Nursing Research, 24,* 324–333.

Krehbiel, R., Munsick-Bruno, G., & Lowe, J. R. (1991). NICU infants at developmental risk and the individualized family service plan/process (IFSP). *Children's Health Care, 20,* 26–33.

Kuhn, T. (1970). *The structure of scientific revolutions* (2nd ed.). Chicago: University of Chicago Press.

McBride, S. L., Brotherson, M. J., Joanning, H., Whiddon, D., & Demmitt, A. (1993). Implementation of family-centered services: Perceptions of families and professionals. *Journal of Early Intervention, 17,* 414–430.

McCluskey-Fawcett, K., O'Brien, M., Robinson, P., & Asay, J. H. (1992). Early transitions for the parents of premature infants: Implications for intervention. *Infant Mental Health Journal, 13,* 147–156.

Mehren, E. (1991). *Born too soon.* New York: Doubleday.

Minde, K., Shosenberg, N., Marton, P., Thompson, J., Ripley, J., & Burns, S. (1980). Self-help groups in a premature nursery: A controlled evaluation. *Journal of Pediatrics, 96,* 933–939.

Miller, M., Mutton, C., & Williams, B. F. (1993). Collaborated experiences for NICU and early childhood education personnel. *Neonatal Network, 12,* 37–42.

Minuchin, S. (1974). *Families and family therapy.* Cambridge, MA: Howard University Press.

Nathanson, M. (1986). *Organizing and maintaining support groups for parents with chronic illness and handicapping conditions.* Washington, DC: Association for the Care of Children's Health.

NEC*TAS and ACCH. (1989). *Guidelines and recommended practices for the individualized family service plan.* Washington, DC: National Early Childhood Technical Assistance System and Association for the Care of Children's Health.

O'Brien, M., & Dale, D. (1994). Family-centered services in the neonatal intensive care unit: A review of research. *Journal of Early Intervention, 18,* 79–90.

Oster, A. (1984). Keynote address for comprehensive approaches to disabled and at-risk infants, toddlers and their families. In *Equals in this partnership: Parents of disabled and at-risk infants speak to professionals* (pp 26–32). Washington, DC: Maternal and Child Health Clearing House.

Parker, S. J., Zahr, L. K., Cole, J. G., & Brecht, M. (1992). Outcome after developmental intervention in the neonatal intensive care unit for mothers of preterm infants with low socioeconomic status. *Journal of Pediatrics, 120,* 780–785.

Plass, K. (1994). The evolution of parental roles in the NICU. *Neonatal Network, 13,* 31–33.

Rushton, C. H. (1990). Family-centered care in the critical care setting: Myth or reality? *Children's Health Care, 19,* 68–78.

Scarr-Salapatek, S., & Williams, M. L. (1973). The effects of early stimulation on low birthweight infants. *Child Development, 44,* 94–101.

Shelton, T., Jeppson, E., & Johnson, B (1987). *Family-centered care for children with special health care needs.* Washington, DC: Association for the Care of Children's Health.

Thurman, S. K., Cornwell, J. R., & Korteland, C. (1989). The Liaison Infant Family Team (LIFT) Project: An example of case study evaluation. *Infants and Young Children, 2,* 74–82.

Thurman, S. K., & Korteland, C. (1989). The behavior of mothers and fathers toward their infants during neonatal intensive care visits. *Children's Health Care, 18*, 247–251.

Thurman, S. K. (1991). Parameters for establishing family-centered neonatal intensive care services. *Children's Health Care, 20*, 34–39.

Thurman, S. K. (1993). Intervention in the neonatal intensive care unit. In W. Brown, S. K. Thurman, & L. F. Pearl (Eds.), *Family-centered early intervention with infants & toddlers: Innovative cross-disciplinary approach* (pp. 173–209). Baltimore, MD: Paul H. Brookes Publishing.

Turnbull, A. P., & Summers, J. A. (1985, April). *From parent involvement to family support: Evolution to revolution.* Paper presented at the Down syndrome State-of-the-Art Conference. Boston, MA.

Turnbull, A. P., & Turnbull, H. R. (1986). *Families, professionals and exceptionality: A special partnership.* Columbus, OH.: Merrill Publishing.

VandenBerg, K. (1987). Revising the traditional model: An individualized approach to developmental interventions in the intensive care nursery. *Neonatal Network, 3*, 32–38.

VandenBerg, K., & Hanson, M. J. (1993). *Homecoming for babies after the neonatal intensive care nursery: A guide for professionals in supporting families and their infants' early development.* Austin, TX: Pro-Ed.

Vestal, K. W., & Richardson, K. (1981). The nature of pediatric critical care nursing: Perspectives of patient, family and staff. *Nursing Clinics of North America, 16*, 605–610.

Watterson-Wells, P., DeBoard-Burns, M. B., Cook, R. C., & Mitchell, J. (1994). Growing up in the hospital: Part II, Nurturing the philosophy of family-centered care. *Journal of Pediatric Nursing, 9*, 141–149.

White, J. L., & Labarba, R. C. (1976). The effects of tactile and kinesthetic stimulation on neonatal development in the premature infant. *Developmental Psychology, 9*, 569–577.

Widmayer, S. M., & Field, T. M. (1981). Effects of Brazelton demonstrations for mothers in the development of preterm infants. *Pediatrics, 67*, 711–714.

Winch, E., & Christoph, J. M. (1988). Parent-to-parent links: Building networks for parents of hospitalized children. *Children's Health Care, 17*, 93–97.

Wyly, V., & Allen, J. (1990). *Stress and coping in the NICU.* Tucson, AZ: Communication Skill Builders.

Wyly, V. (1993, March). *Family-centered care in the NICU: Training NICU health providers and early interventionists.* Paper presented at National Parent Care Conference, San Francisco, CA.

Wyly, M. V., Allen, J., Pfalzer, S., & Wilson, J. R. (1993, December). *Linking NICU health providers and early interventionists for family-centered care.* Paper presented at the National Center for Clinical Infant Programs, Washington, DC.

INDEX

■